MOVE BETTER, FEEL BETTER

CHAIR EXERCISES

FOR SENIORS OVER 60

Linette Cunley

DISCLAIMER

The information in this book is provided for educational and entertainment purposes only. Every effort has been made to present accurate, up-to-date, and reliable information. However, no warranties of any kind are expressed or implied. The author does not offer legal, financial, medical, or professional advice. Readers are strongly encouraged to consult a licensed professional before attempting any of the techniques described in this book.

HEALTH AND SAFETY NOTICE

This book is not intended to diagnose, treat, cure, or prevent any medical condition. The information provided is for educational purposes only and should not be considered medical advice. Always consult with a qualified healthcare professional before beginning any exercise program or implementing any suggestions from this book, especially if you have pre-existing conditions, injuries, or concerns about your physical or mental health. The author and publisher are not responsible for any health-related issues that may arise from the use of the information in this book.

By reading this book, the reader agrees that the author and publisher are not responsible for any losses, injuries, or issues that may result from the application of the information herein, including but not limited to errors, omissions, or inaccuracies.

TABLE OF CONTENTS

TABLE OF CONTENTS

INTRODUCTION

Chair exercises provide a safe, low-cost, and accessible practice for seniors to benefit from physical activity. The benefits of this exercise method are numerous and include improving and maintaining strength for older adults (Klempel et al., 2021). A challenging and well-rounded chair exercise program can also improve your balance and mobility, and increase your stamina and confidence.

This book is designed for older adults who wish to be active in a way that's safe, effective, and practical. These chair exercises can be done in the comfort of your home with minimal equipment required. The exercises presented in this book are meant for all fitness levels. Whether you're recovering from an injury, dealing with arthritis, or simply looking for a gentle workout, you will be able to adapt these exercises to your needs.

TIPS FOR GETTING STARTED

Getting started and staying consistent are the most challenging parts of any fitness journey. However, once you build momentum, we hope that you create a healthy habit for life. Here are a few tips to help you take the first steps:

Set realistic goals: Set health goals that are realistic and aligned with your needs. We will discuss how to establish SMART goals later in the guide.

Show up consistently: There are days when you will feel motivated to exercise and other days when you will feel like giving up. What's important is to show up consistently to create a habit. Remember that doing something is better than doing nothing. A helpful tip is the 10-minute rule. Tell yourself you will exercise for 10 minutes and if it doesn't feel good, you can stop. The chances are, once you start you will feel much better and will be able to keep going.

Embrace the discomfort: When you are exercising and finding your body is being challenged, see this as a positive sign. You will get stronger and more fit with each practice session, so just stay with it and be consistent in your efforts, even on the difficult days.

Listen to your body: Discomfort is necessary for growth, but this doesn't mean you should be in pain or on the brink of exhaustion. Always listen to your body and don't be afraid to modify or stop an exercise if it doesn't feel right for you.

Add it to your schedule: If exercising is not scheduled into your day, it will likely stay on the back burner. How many times do we say, "I'll just do it tomorrow"? Six months down the line, tomorrow never comes. With the structured plan provided in this book, it will be easier to input each workout into your schedule. Consider "bundling" your exercise by scheduling it right after something else that you already do every day, so that you remember it is time to workout. For instance, you might schedule your workout right after you have a cup of coffee, or walk the dog; that way, you'll find it easier to remember when it is time to practice your chair exercises.

SAFETY PRECAUTIONS

Safety should always come first. Here are the main safety precautions to consider when you are practicing chair exercises:

- **Consult your healthcare provider**: Before starting any new fitness program, check with your doctor. If you haven't had a health check in a while, we definitely recommend getting one to make sure you can safely exercise.

- **Stay hydrated**: Keep water nearby and take breaks as needed.

- **Follow breathing cues**: Don't hold your breath while exercising. Maintain a steady breathing pattern, particularly if you have a known cardiovascular condition or high blood pressure. Specific breathing cues are given in each section containing the exercises.

- **Keep a phone nearby**: Although chair exercises are safe, emergencies can still happen. Keep a phone nearby in case you need to call for help and if you share your living space, inform those around you about your planned activity so they can assist if needed.

We discuss specific safety precautions in more detail later. In the next chapter, we dive deeper into the benefits of chair exercises and dispel common myths about this way of exercising.

UNDERSTANDING CHAIR EXERCISES

Chair exercises provide a simple way to exercise but can have a significant impact on your health and quality of life. Chair exercises can be performed by individuals of all ages; they are especially well-suited for seniors because they offer a safe and low-impact alternative to traditional workouts. Let's explore why they are effective, and address some of the common misconceptions.

BENEFITS OF CHAIR EXERCISES

Below are some of the main benefits of chair exercises that have been documented (Klempel et al., 2021; Mackie & Eng, 2023; Platz et al., 2023):

Increased Strength: Targeted chair exercises can help to build lower and upper body muscles, as well as core strength.

Improved Mobility: Gentle stretching can give you a better sense of ease in your everyday movements.

Improved Heart Health: Chair exercises allow for a low-impact option for cardiovascular activity. Although this area requires more research, patients with cardiovascular conditions respond well to chair-based exercises for rehabilitation.

Better Balance: Exercises that strengthen your core and challenge your balance help reduce the risk of falls. Consequently, you can also reduce the risk of injury and improve your confidence during daily activities.

Psychological Improvements: A regular chair-based exercise routine can have a positive impact on psychological health. One of the main appeals of this simple exercise method is to reconnect with the joy of movement without the fear of injury or exhaustion.

CHAIR EXERCISE VS. OTHER EXERCISE

Each type of exercise comes with its unique set of benefits and limitations. Chair exercises are sometimes preferred to others, especially for seniors and individuals with limited mobility or balance.

Let's compare chair exercises to some of the main forms of exercise to better understand the advantages.

Standing Exercises: Standing exercises can pose a significant risk for safety for seniors with balance issues. Chair exercises provide increased stability whether this means physically sitting on the chair or using the chair as support in a standing position.

High-Impact Workouts: Activities like running, jogging, or even dancing are considered high-impact, which can be great for getting your heart rate up and improving your overall cardiovascular health, but strenuous on the joints. Alternatively, low-impact cardiovascular exercises can be performed with the use of a chair. You will still be able to get your heart rate up with less stress on your lower back, hips, knees, and ankles.

Mat-Based Workouts: Pilates, yoga, and floor stretches are some examples of mat-based workouts. They are excellent for improving flexibility and strength. The only problem is, they require getting up and down from the floor. Chair exercises ensure you stay comfortable the entire time you exercise.

Gym-Based Workouts: Gym workouts allow you to have access to a lot of equipment, but they are often costly and involve you going out of your way which can be a barrier to regular exercise. Chair exercises can be done in the comfort of your home, so you have higher chances of staying consistent.

COMMON MYTHS AND FACTS

It's not uncommon to have preconceived ideas about something you've never tried before. If you're reading this, you have probably already decided to give chair exercises a chance. If you're still skeptical about the benefits of chair exercises, perhaps the following myths and facts will convince you otherwise.

Myth 1: Chair exercises are just for "old people."

Fact: Chair-based exercises are a proven and effective way to stay active at any age. Chair exercises are beneficial for seniors and individuals with limited balance and mobility, but others benefit from it too. Office workers often use chair-based exercises to alleviate tension from prolonged sitting postures during the work day, and injured athletes incorporate more chair-based exercises into their regimen when they have a restriction on weight-bearing activities.

Myth 2: Chair exercises are boring.

Fact: Any workout can be as fun as you make it. Try varying the workouts, taking a playful approach, and playing music to make the experience more enjoyable.

Myth 3: You can't do chair exercises if you already have another exercise routine.

Fact: Chair exercises can be done as a standalone practice or as a complement to any existing workout routine. Be sure to allow proper recovery between strenuous routines and try to include light to moderate-intensity activities like walking or swimming in your exercise regimen on top of the chair-based exercise.

Myth 4: Chair exercises are too easy to be effective.

Fact: The effectiveness of chair exercises has been documented. Know that you can always adjust the intensity to match your current fitness level. This can be done by adding more resistance, increasing the speed, or performing more sets and repetitions.

Myth 5: You need expensive equipment.

Fact: Many chair exercises simply use body weight. They sometimes require equipment, like elastic bands and light weights, but the cost of these is minimal. Plus, most of the equipment required for chair-based exercises can be substituted for household items.

Chair exercises are versatile enough to meet you where you are while allowing you to gradually improve your health and fitness. Whether you're using them as a starting point or a supplement to other workouts, they're a safe and efficient tool for maintaining an active lifestyle.

GETTING READY

2

Let's make sure you are set up for success before you start performing the chair-based exercises included in this book. We'll go over selecting the right chair, creating a safe workout environment, and gathering any necessary equipment.

CHOOSING THE RIGHT CHAIR

Your chair is the foundation of your workout and selecting the right one will allow for maximum comfort. These are the main features your chair should have:

Stability: Select a chair with a sturdy and even base. Avoid chairs with wheels.

Height and depth: When seated comfortably on the chair, your feet should rest on the floor. Make sure your circulation is not being cut off at the back of your knees.

Support: The optimal chair should have a comfortable and supportive backrest at about the height of your shoulder blades.

Armrests: A chair without armrests will allow more range of motion. For individuals requiring more assistance to get in and out of the chair, one with armrests might be preferable.

CREATING A SAFE WORKOUT SPACE

The environment that you exercise in should feel comfortable and inviting. Clear the area around your chair to prevent tripping hazards. You should be able to comfortably stretch your arms out to the sides. You can place a yoga mat under the chair for non-slip protection. You should also select a space where you have access to an uncluttered wall as some of the exercises require propping the chair against a wall.

The lighting can be soft and soothing to promote a sense of wellbeing. You can add candles or plants for a relaxing effect, and adjust the room temperature if you start getting too warm or too cold.

EQUIPMENT

Resistance Bands: These are inexpensive, lightweight, and easy to store. They also come with different levels of resistance which allows you to increase resistance as you improve. These can be used for upper and lower-body resistance training.

Light Weights: Small dumbbells are great for upper-body chair exercises. If you don't have dumbbells, you can use water bottles or canned goods. One of the self-assessments in Chapter 11 requires a 5-pound dumbbell for women and an 8-pound dumbbell for men. This is a good place to start for upper-body exercises; as you improve you can always purchase heavier dumbbells as needed.

Velcro weights can be useful for upper-body strengthening, especially for individuals who struggle to hold a weight in their hands. In this case, they can be placed around the wrist. They can also be used instead of resistance bands for the lower-body strengthening chair exercises.

Flexibility accessories: Yoga straps are useful for exercises like seated calf stretches or seated quad stretches. They provide support and allow for a more comfortable stretch. If you don't have a yoga strap, you can also use a belt, towel, or scarf.

Miscellaneous accessories: A small towel can come in handy if you sweat during your workout. A water bottle can help you stay hydrated during your workout. A cushion can increase comfort in your buttock region area during seated chair exercises. Some individuals might also like to place a cushion between the backrest and their back during some seated positions.

MODIFYING EXERCISES FOR COMFORT

Exercise modifications and adaptations ensure that you feel comfortable and confident in performing the chair exercises. Most of the exercises presented in this book are in a seated position. However, there are a select few described in a standing position with the assistance of the chair. Always make sure the chair is safely propped up against the wall for maximum safety while you use it for support. You can also stand in front of a kitchen counter for these exercises if your space allows it. If you're feeling insecure about performing the standing exercises unsupervised, stick to the ones in a seated position.

Never force a joint to move past its available range or a muscle to stretch beyond its limits. Start with the range of motion that is available and comfortable for you. As you get more flexible, progressively increase the range.

It's possible that you may find your strength is very limited for a specific strength exercise. If this happens, try your best and perform as many repetitions as you can. Start with body weight and increase the number of repetitions as you get stronger. Eventually, you will be able to add some light weight to the movement.

Start Small: If you're new to exercise or are coming back to it after a long break, take it easy. Start by performing the movements in a smaller range of motion. Once you feel more confident in your abilities, increase the range.

Use Props: As you have probably noticed, some exercises involve using a towel or a yoga strap to assist with working on flexibility. Don't be afraid to use these as they can reduce the strain on your joints and make the stretch more comfortable. Another prop that can be used is a cushion to increase comfort during the chair exercises. You can place the cushion under your seat to add padding or you could also place it behind your lower back to encourage a comfortable upright posture.

Adapt the Duration: If an exercise session feels too long or strenuous for your fitness level, there is no shame in cutting it short. You could still perform the entire workout for that day by doing it in bite-size pieces. This might make it feel more manageable for beginners and reduce fatigue.

CONSIDERATION FOR SPECIFIC CONDITIONS

In this section, we go over some of the main conditions that need to be considered when exercising, and suggest some modifications you can do instead (Chilibeck et al., 2011). If you have any health related questions, please consult with your doctor.

Arthritis

Arthritis is a general term that means inflammation of the joints. There are many different forms of arthritis including rheumatoid arthritis, ankylosing spondylitis, and psoriatic arthritis, to name a few examples. These can vary in severity from person to person. Physical activity is encouraged for individuals affected by arthritis. That being said, you may need to modify their routine, especially when you are experiencing a flare-up. The goal is to keep the joints strong and mobile without adding to the inflammation. For individuals with advanced forms of arthritis, heavy load-bearing exercises are not recommended. Luckily, non-weight-bearing exercises, like chair exercises, are safe.

You may need to adapt the time at which you do your exercises depending on your symptoms. Individuals with arthritis are usually stiffer in the morning. It might be advisable to perform your exercises when the joints feel less stiff. Make sure you respect your symptoms as you exercise. Even though chair exercises are safe for people with arthritis, don't push through a movement if it doesn't feel comfortable for a specific joint.

Osteoporosis

Osteoporosis is a condition in which the bone mass is decreased. This happens as we age, and women are more affected than men due to hormonal changes with menopause. Due to the bones being more brittle, it can lead to an increased risk of fracture. Exercise is recommended for individuals with osteoporosis; it can actually stimulate bone regeneration. However, we want to minimize the fracture risk while exercising.

Trunk flexion exercises (forward bend) should be avoided if you are at high risk of fracture. Individuals who have had previous fractures resulting from weak bones or who have been taking corticosteroids (prednisone-equivalent dose $\geq$7.5 mg daily) for three months or more within the last year are considered high risk. Forceful twisting motions of the trunk should be avoided. Start with a light to moderate intensity when exercising and progress depending on your abilities. During exercises that require twisting motions of the trunk, go very slowly or substitute with another exercise of your choice.

During trunk flexion exercises, avoid rounding the spine by keeping a bend in your knees and hinging at the hips instead. If you have doubts about the safety of a specific exercise you can always skip it or substitute it with another exercise of your choice.

Lower Back Pain

Low back pain is complex and can vary greatly depending on the individual. We know that an integral part of treating low back pain is physical activity. What's recommended is to exercise while respecting the symptoms. When you are in intense and acute pain, high-impact exercise and heavy resistance training should be avoided. It's also recommended to stay away from any extreme trunk flexion, extension, or rotation that reproduces intense pain.

Exercise as tolerated with low back pain. A good rule of thumb is assessing your pain on a scale of 1-10, 10 being the worst pain you have ever felt. If you perform a movement and your pain is at a 3 out of 10 or less, you are in the safe zone. If you have undergone back surgery or have a more severe condition involving nerve compression, for example, make sure you consult with your healthcare provider for tailored advice.

Avoid poses that bring the head below the heart if you have high blood pressure, glaucoma, dizziness, or vertigo. Avoid extreme side bends of the trunk if you have recently suffered an injury to your ribs. If you have diabetes, make sure you keep a snack nearby and monitor blood sugar levels before and after exercise. It's always better to respect your individual needs instead of pushing through something that doesn't feel right.

WARM-UP AND COOL-DOWN

3

THE BENEFITS OF WARMING UP

Starting an exercise session with a warm-up creates several beneficial physiological changes. In other words, warming up impacts your body's natural functions. First, warming up increases blood circulation, supplying more oxygen to the muscles and nerves. This will allow your muscles to contract more efficiently and improve the signals sent from the nerves to the muscles. This way, you will have better coordination and control during your workout.

Next, warming up also increases body temperature. During exercise, our body will naturally have to increase its body temperature. Therefore, the warm-up ensures a gradual transition. You should warm up at a low intensity to avoid overexerting yourself from the start. Spend a few minutes warming up with slow, gentle movements before transitioning into the more demanding part of your workout.

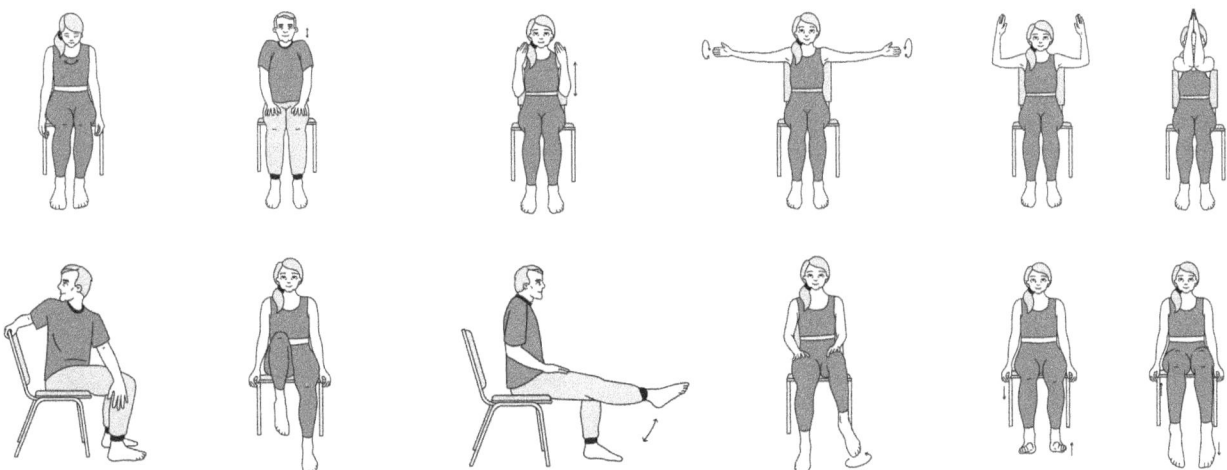

WARM-UP ROUTINE

NECK ROLLS

Focus: Neck muscles and joints.

- Sit upright with your feet flat on the floor.

- Slowly drop your chin towards your chest, then gently roll your head to the right, bringing your ear toward your shoulder.

- Then, bring your head back to the center and your head to the left.

- Continue to roll your head in a half circle from the right to the left about ten times.

Breathing: Maintain steady breathing throughout the exercise.

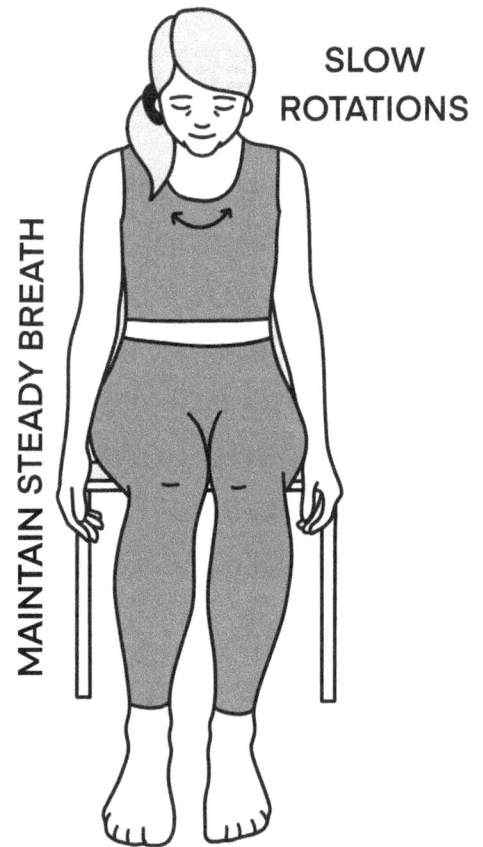

SLOW ROTATIONS

MAINTAIN STEADY BREATH

SHOULDER SHRUGS

Focus: Shoulder and lower neck muscles.

- Sit upright and relax your arms by your side.

- Gently shrug your shoulders towards your ears.

- Hold at the top for a moment, then release the shoulders.

- Repeat ten times.

Breathing: Inhale as you lift the shoulders, and exhale as you release.

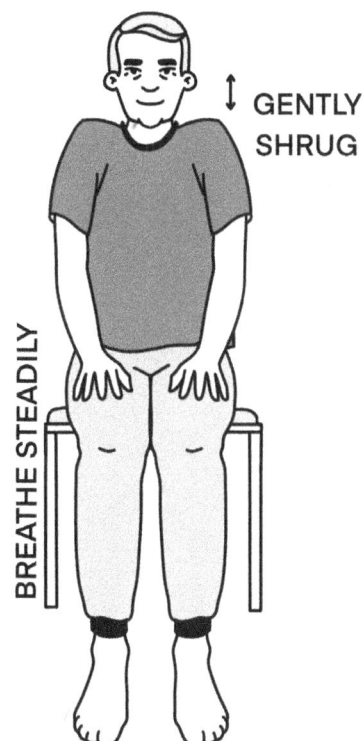

GENTLY SHRUG

BREATHE STEADILY

BENDING AND EXTENDING ELBOWS

Focus: Elbow joints and muscles.

- Sit upright with your arms by your sides.

- Slowly bend your elbows to bring your hands toward your shoulders, then release your arms back down.

- Repeat ten times.

Breathing: Inhale as you bend your elbows, and exhale as you extend.

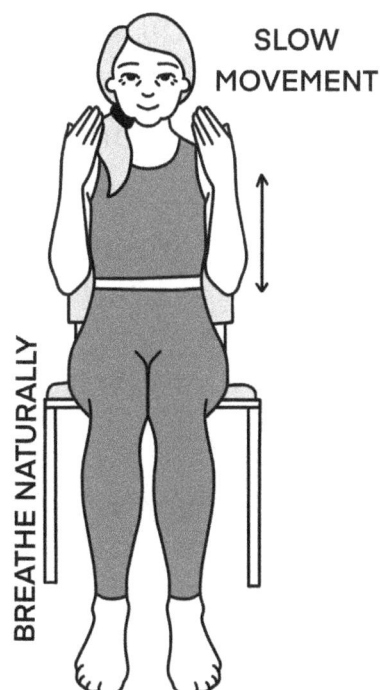

SLOW MOVEMENT

BREATHE NATURALLY

ARM CIRCLES

SLOW ROTATION

STEADY BREATHING

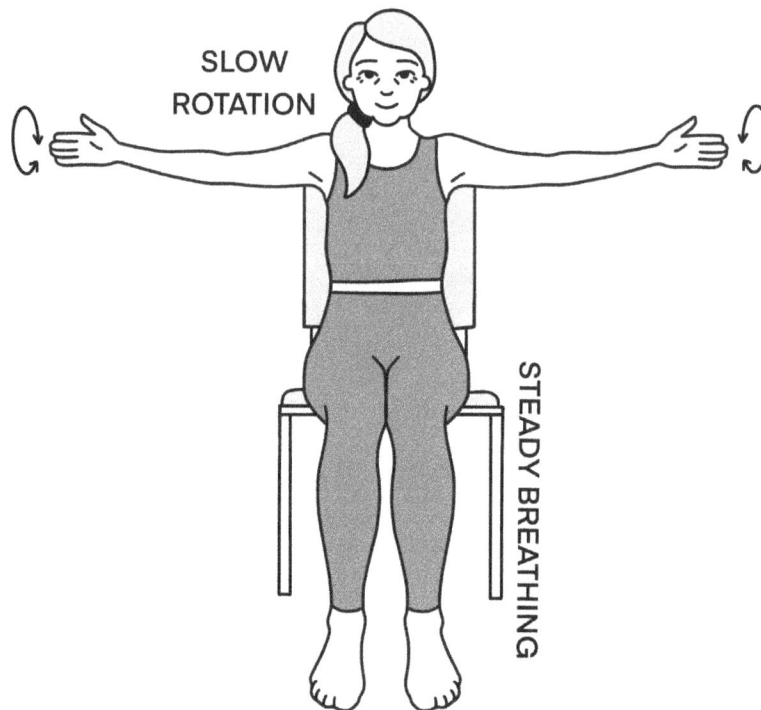

Focus: Shoulder joints.

- Sit upright with your feet flat on the floor.
- Extend both arms out to the sides at shoulder height.
- Make small circles with your arms, rotating them forward for ten repetitions, then rotating backward for another ten repetitions.

Breathing: Maintain steady breathing throughout the entire exercise.

SEATED CHEST OPENER

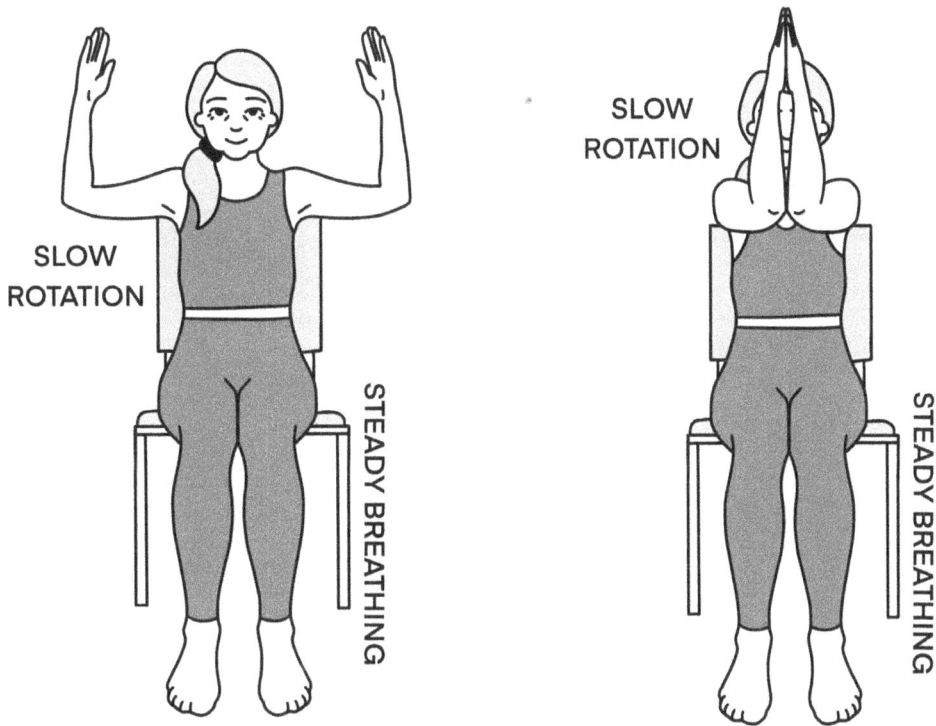

SLOW ROTATION

SLOW ROTATION

STEADY BREATHING

SLOW ROTATION

STEADY BREATHING

Focus: Chest muscles and upper-back and shoulder joints.

- Sit upright in the chair with your feet flat on the floor.
- Bring both arms in cactus position with elbows and shoulders at a 90-degree angle.
- Arch your back and open your chest as you reach your arms backward.
- Then, gently round your back as you bring your palms and forearms to touch. (Your arms should remain at shoulder height.)
- Slowly move back and forth ten times.

Breathing: Inhale as you arch your back and exhale as you round your back.

SEATED TWIST

Focus: Muscles and joints of the entire spine.

- Sit tall with your feet hip-width apart and flat on the ground.
- Place your right hand on the outside of your left knee, and your left hand behind you on the chair.
- Slowly twist your torso to the left, looking over your left shoulder.
- Come back to center and repeat on the other side. Repeat five times on each side.

Breathing: Inhale as you lengthen your spine in the center and exhale as you twist.

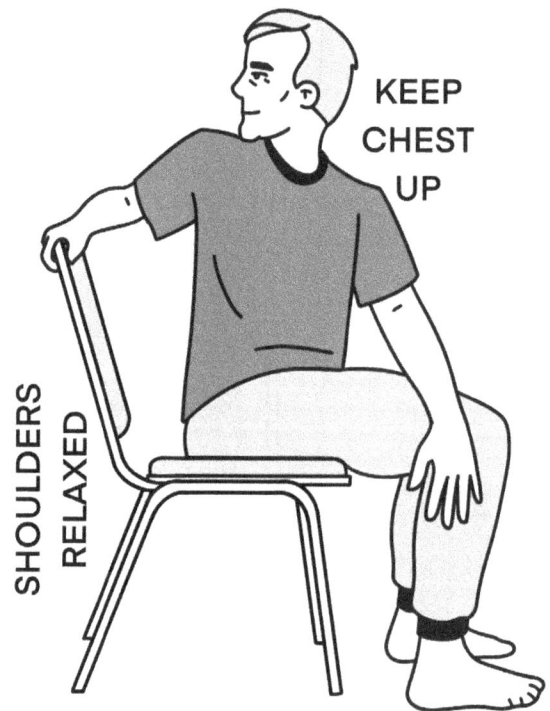

KEEP CHEST UP

SHOULDERS RELAXED

SEATED MARCHES

Focus: Hip muscles and joints as well as core muscles.

- Sit tall with your feet flat on the ground.

- Lift one knee toward your chest, as if you're marching in place while seated.

- Lower that leg and lift the other knee toward your chest.

- Alternate knees, ten times on each side.

Breathing: Inhale as you lift your leg, then exhale as you lower it.

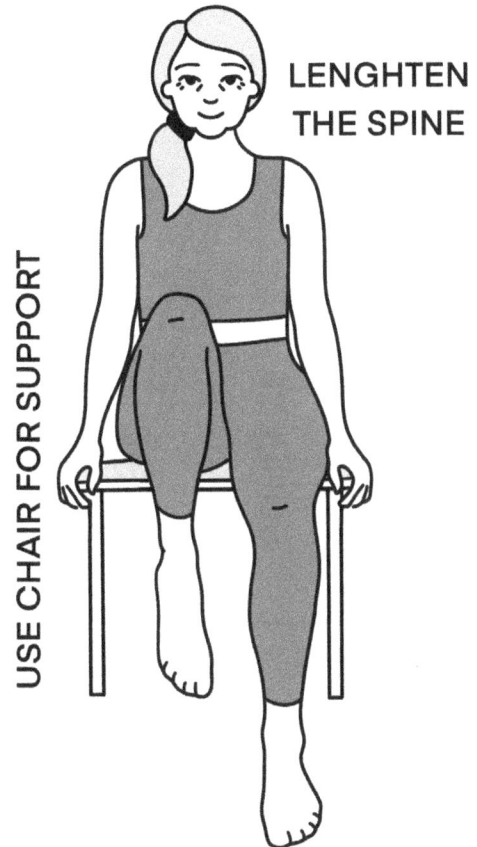

LENGHTEN THE SPINE

USE CHAIR FOR SUPPORT

SEATED LEG EXTENSIONS

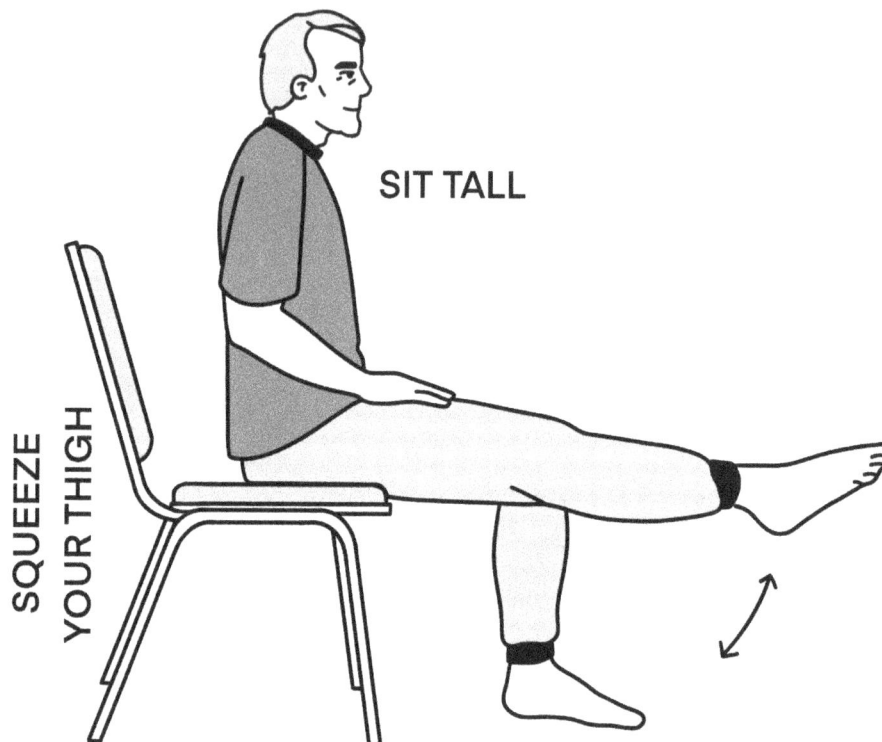

SIT TALL

SQUEEZE YOUR THIGH

Focus: Knee and quadricep muscles.

- Sit tall with your feet flat on the floor.

- Slowly extend your right leg out in front of you. (It is okay if you can't fully straighten the knee.) Squeeze your thigh muscle and hold for a moment before releasing your leg.

- Repeat with the left leg, then alternate ten times on each side.

Breathing: Maintain steady breathing throughout this exercise.

ANKLE CIRCLES

Focus: Ankle joints and muscles.

- Sit tall with your feet flat on the floor.

- Lift one foot slightly off the floor and begin to rotate your ankle in a circle.

- Repeat ten times clockwise and ten times counterclockwise.

- Release your leg back down and repeat the same thing on the other side.

Breathing: Maintain steady breathing throughout this exercise.

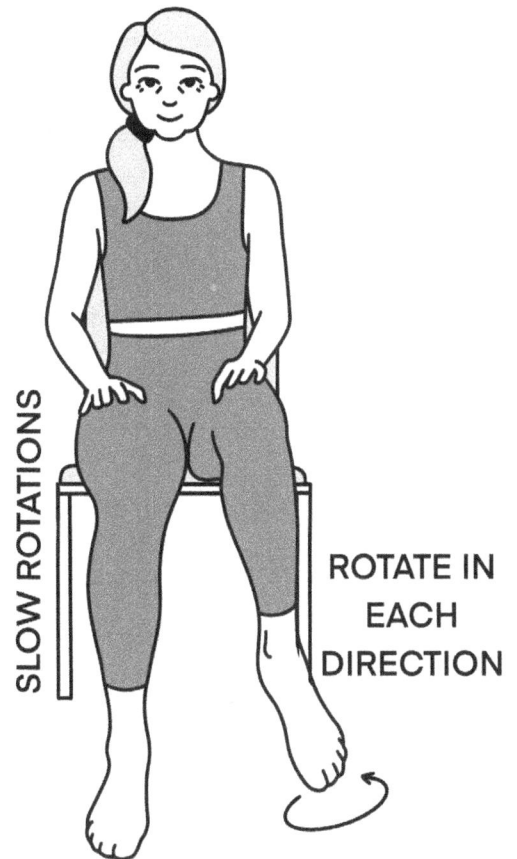

SLOW ROTATIONS

ROTATE IN EACH DIRECTION

HEEL-TOE TAPS

SIT TALL

USE CHAIR FOR SUPPORT

MAINTAIN STEADY BREATHING

FLEX YOUR CALVES

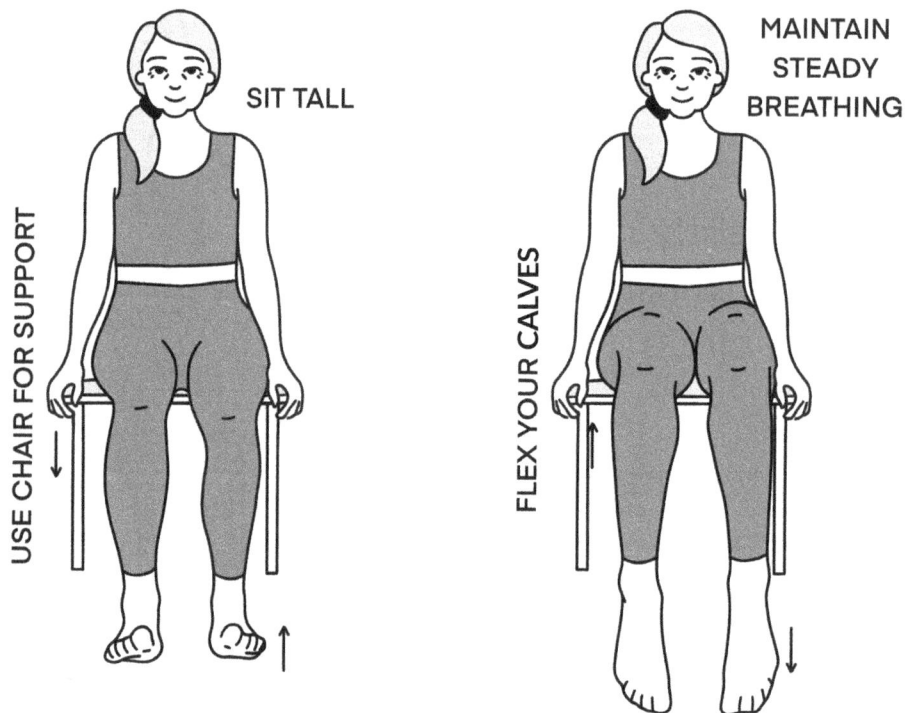

Focus: Ankle joints, calves, and shins.

- Sit tall with your feet flat on the floor.

- Lift the toes of both feet off the floor while keeping your heels planted, then, lower the toes back down.

- Next, lift your heels off the ground by pushing through the balls of your feet, then, lower the heels back down.

- Alternate between lifting your toes and your heels for 20 repetitions.

Breathing: Maintain steady breathing throughout this exercise.

BENEFITS OF COOLING DOWN

We've highlighted the importance of warming up before exercise, but cooling down also has its benefits, including gradually lowering your heart rate (especially after more intense cardio routines), supporting recovery by allowing the body to rest and repair, and promoting mental well-being. This last benefit will allow you to feel the emotional benefits of exercise, such as a better mood and an increased sense of well-being and gratitude.

The great thing about a cool-down is that it doesn't need to take long to be effective. Just five minutes at the end of a workout can help bring your heart rate back to normal. In fact, studies suggest to keep cool-downs under thirty minutes, because a longer cool-down could potentially interfere with your body's ability to replenish your energy stores, or glycogen (Van Hooren, B., & Peake, J. M. (2018).

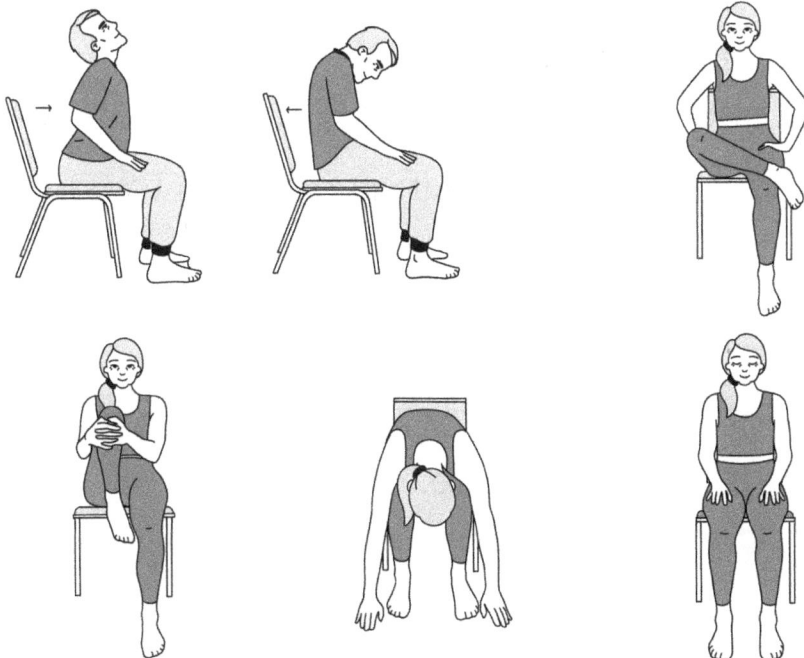

COOL-DOWN ROUTINE

SEATED CAT-COW STRETCH

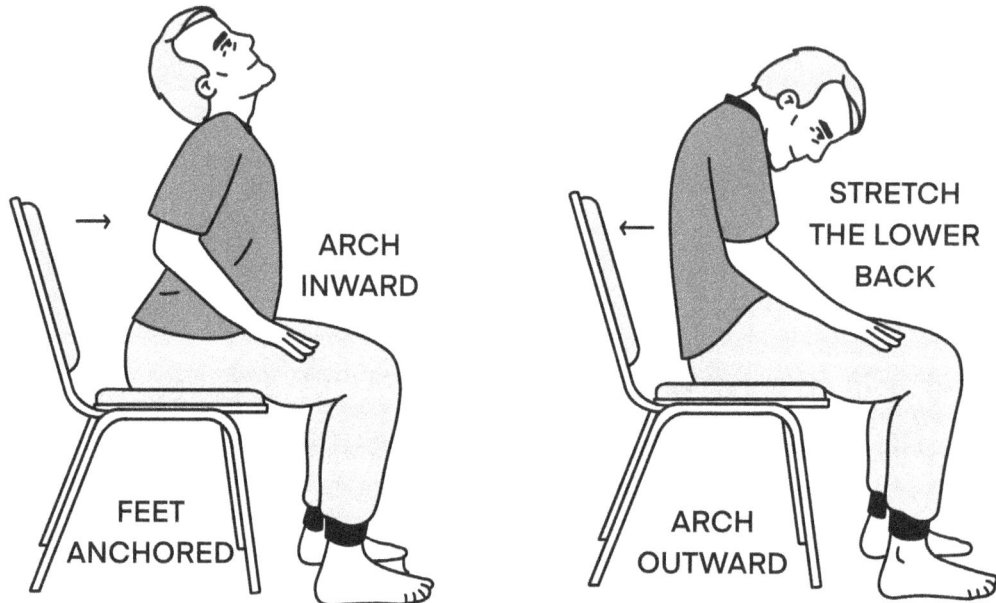

ARCH INWARD

FEET ANCHORED

STRETCH THE LOWER BACK

ARCH OUTWARD

Focus: Vertebral column joints.

- Sit tall with your feet flat on the ground.

- Place your hands on your knees.

- Inhale to arch your back and look slightly upward (cow pose).

- Then, exhale to round your back, tucking your chin toward your chest (cat pose).

- Slowly repeat this movement ten times.

Breathing: Inhale as you arch your back into cow pose, and exhale as you round into cat pose.

FIGURE-4 STRETCH

Focus: Hip joints and muscles.

- Sit tall with your feet flat on the floor.

- Cross your right ankle over your left knee to create a figure-4 shape.

- Keep your back straight or gently lean your torso forward to increase the stretch.

- If it's comfortable for your hip, gently press down on your right knee to deepen the stretch.

- Hold the position for thirty seconds, then switch sides.

- Repeat a few times on each side.

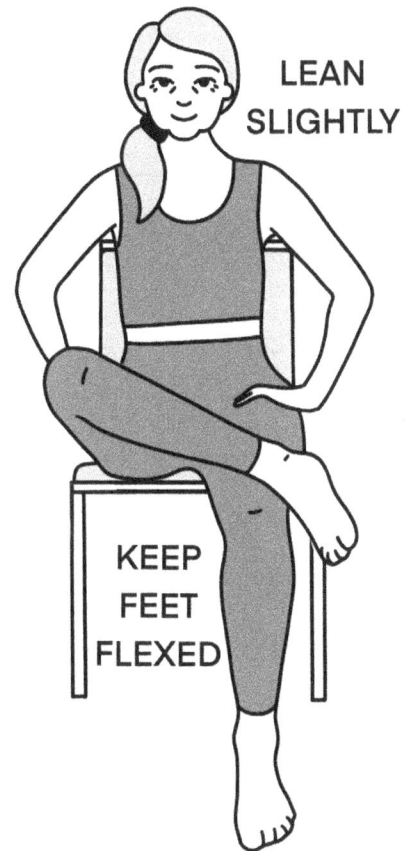

Breathing: Maintain steady breathing throughout the entire movement.

LEAN SLIGHTLY

KEEP FEET FLEXED

HIP FLEXION STRETCH

Focus: Lower back, hip, and knee joints and muscles.

- Sit tall with your back supported.

- Slowly pick up one leg and reach to hold the front of your knee.

- Lift your right knee toward your chest, gently holding it with both hands for support.

- Keep your back straight and avoid rounding the lower back.

- Hold the stretch for thirty seconds, feeling the stretch in your hip and lower back, then release and repeat on the left side.

- Repeat a few times on each side.

AVOID ROUNDING THE LOWER BACK

HOLD KNEE FOR SUPPORT

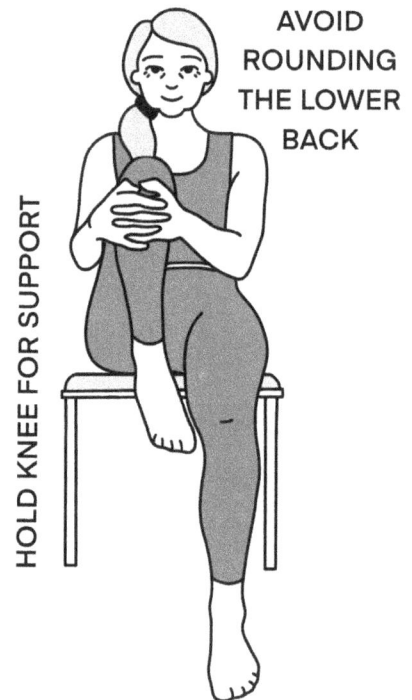

Breathing: Maintain steady breathing throughout the entire movement.

SEATED FORWARD FOLD

Focus: Vertebral column and hamstring muscles.

- Sit on the edge of the chair with your feet flat on the floor at hip-distance apart.

- Slowly fold forward from the hips, reaching your hands toward the floor.

- Relax your head and neck and hold the stretch for thirty seconds.

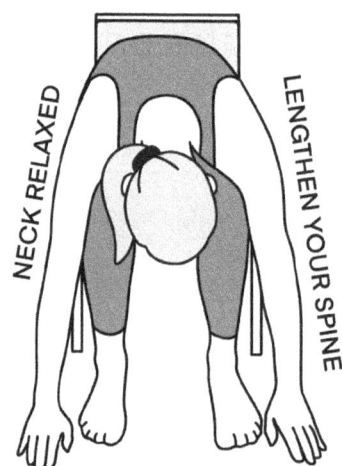

NECK RELAXED

LENGTHEN YOUR SPINE

Breathing: Maintain steady breathing throughout the entire movement.

BOX BREATHING

Focus: Diaphragm muscles (to relax your nervous system).

- Sit comfortably with your feet flat on the floor and your hands resting on your lap.

- Inhale deeply through your nose for four counts, expanding your belly.

- At the top of your inhale, hold your breath for a count of four, then exhale slowly through your mouth for a count of four.

- At the bottom of your exhale, hold your breath for another count of four.

- Repeat this cycle for five breaths.

INHALE DEEPLY

TURN FOCUS INWARD

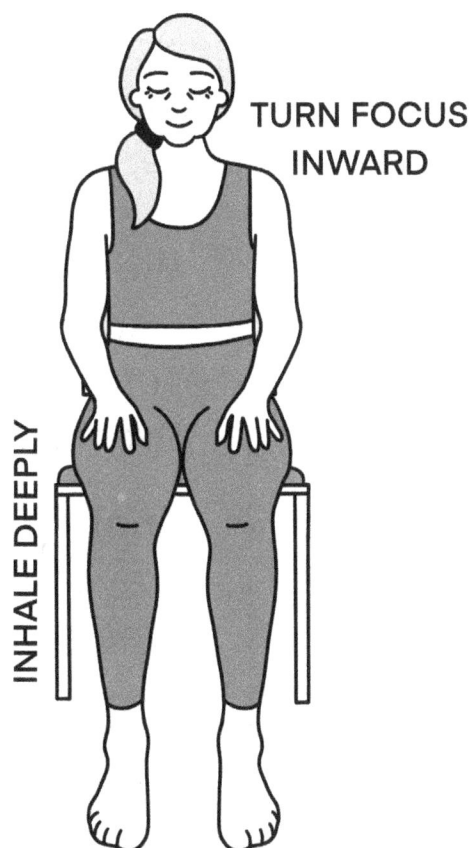

You now have a good base to set you up for success for your warm-ups and cool-downs. In the next chapter, we'll be diving into some chair exercises to strengthen the lower body.

BONUS CONTENT

We want to see you achieve your goals. To help, I've included bonus resources with you in mind: Easy-to-follow Video Tutorials, Printable Trackers, Illustrated Posters and more.

Bonus #1 | **Video Tutorials**
Get Unlimited Access To Easy-To-Follow Video Tutorials That Guide You Through How To Do Every Exercise In The Book.

Bonus #2 | **Printable Trackers And Illustrated Posters**
Stay Motivated And Track Your Progress With Weekly Printable Guides.

Bonus #3 | **7-Step Guide To Kicking Fear And Anxiety**
This Guide Helps You Build Your Confidence And Commit To Establishing A New Wellness Routine.

Bonus #4 | **Guided Meditations**
Immerse Yourself In Calming Guided Meditations Designed To Support Your Wellness Journey.

Bonus #5 | **Facebook Community**
Connect with like-minded individuals, share your progress, ask questions, and receive ongoing support and motivation from both peers and experts.

The **LINK and PIN code to unlock your bonus** is on the **last page of this book**.

These bonuses are **FREE** and **designed to help you achieve your goals**.

UPPER BODY STRENGTH EXERCISES

4

As part of the aging process, we lose strength and muscle mass. Studies have shown that muscle strength decreases by 16.6% to 40.9% in individuals over forty years old (Keller & Engelhardt, 2014). To decrease the effects of muscle loss, it's important to maintain upper body strength. Not only will you feel better, but this will allow you to keep your independence. We need upper-body strength for simple daily activities like carrying groceries or reaching overhead to get something on a shelf. Strong arms, shoulders, chest, and back muscles will help you complete everyday tasks with more confidence and ease.

In this chapter, we'll cover a variety of efficient upper-body exercises. Since these are strengthening exercises, we recommend using some resistance like dumbbells or resistance bands. You can start without resistance to familiarize yourself with the movements, but try to incorporate resistance whenever possible to maximize the effectiveness of the exercise.

EXERCISES FOR ARMS AND SHOULDERS

The arms and shoulders play an important role in everyday movement, from lifting to pushing and pulling. The following exercises target the biceps, triceps, and shoulder muscles. They are meant to help reduce muscle loss and improve strength.

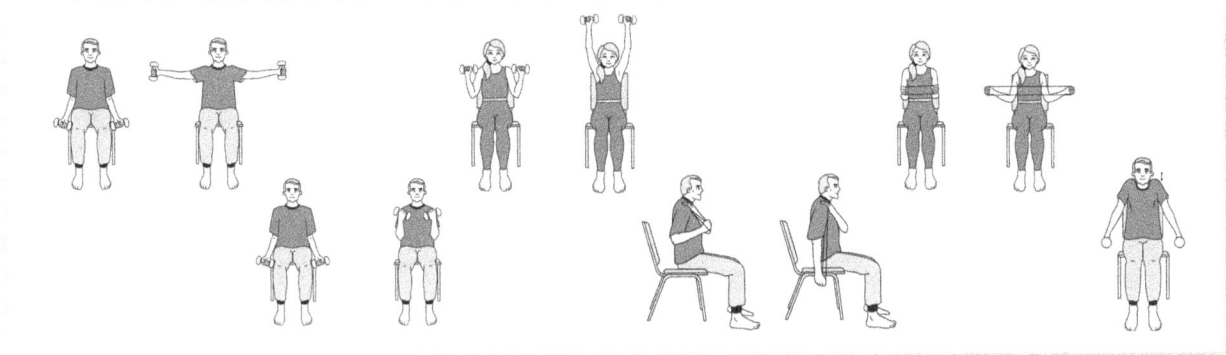

LATERAL RAISES

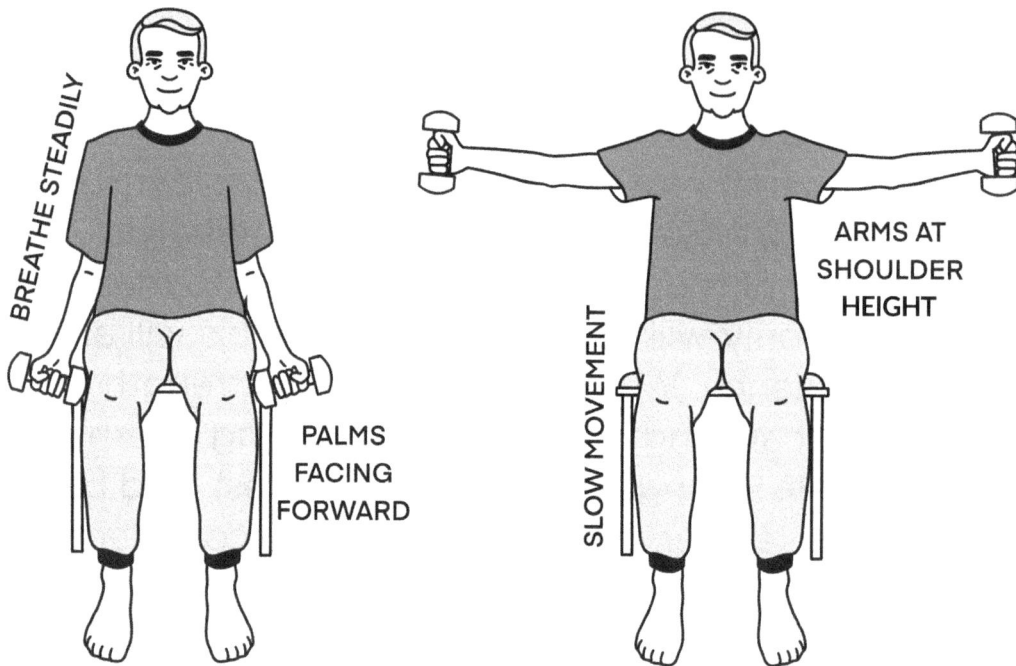

BREATHE STEADILY

PALMS
FACING
FORWARD

SLOW MOVEMENT

ARMS AT
SHOULDER
HEIGHT

Focus: Shoulder muscles, mainly the lateral deltoid.

- Sit tall with your feet flat on the floor.

- Hold a light weight in each hand. (or use wrist Velcro weights).

- With palms facing forward, lift both arms out to the sides at shoulder height, then lower them slowly back to the starting position.

- Perform a few sets of 10-15 repetitions.

Breathing: Exhale as you lift your arms, and inhale as you lower them.

BICEP CURLS

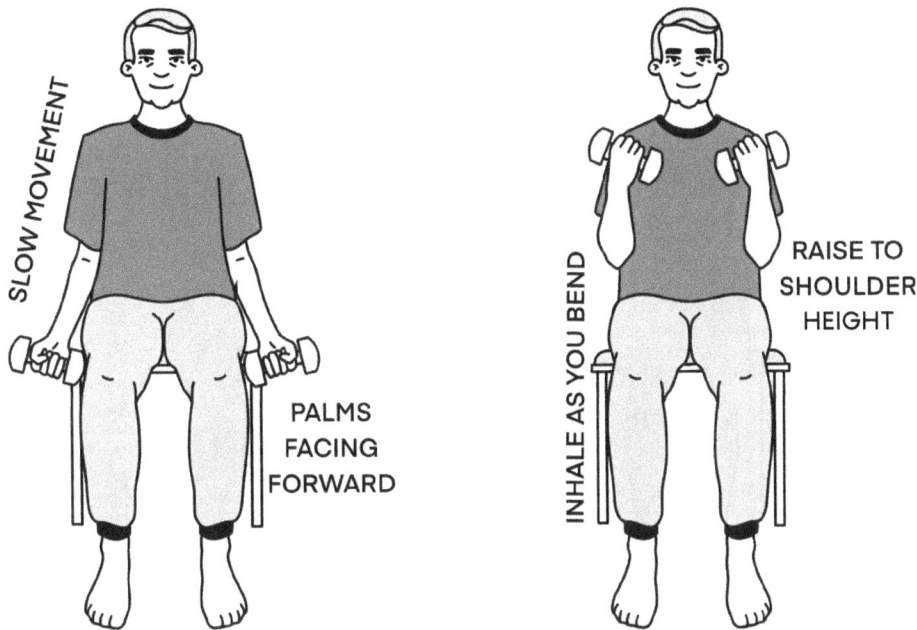

Focus: Biceps muscles.

- Sit tall with your feet flat on the floor.
- Hold a light weight in each hand. You can also use a resistance band by securing one end under your foot on the same side where you are performing the curl.
- Start with your arms at your sides, palms facing forward.
- Slowly bend your elbows to bring the weights toward your shoulders.
- Once you reach the top, lower them back down slowly.
- Perform a few sets of 10-15 repetitions.

Breathing: Inhale as you bend your elbows and exhale as you lower your arms.

SHOULDER PRESSES

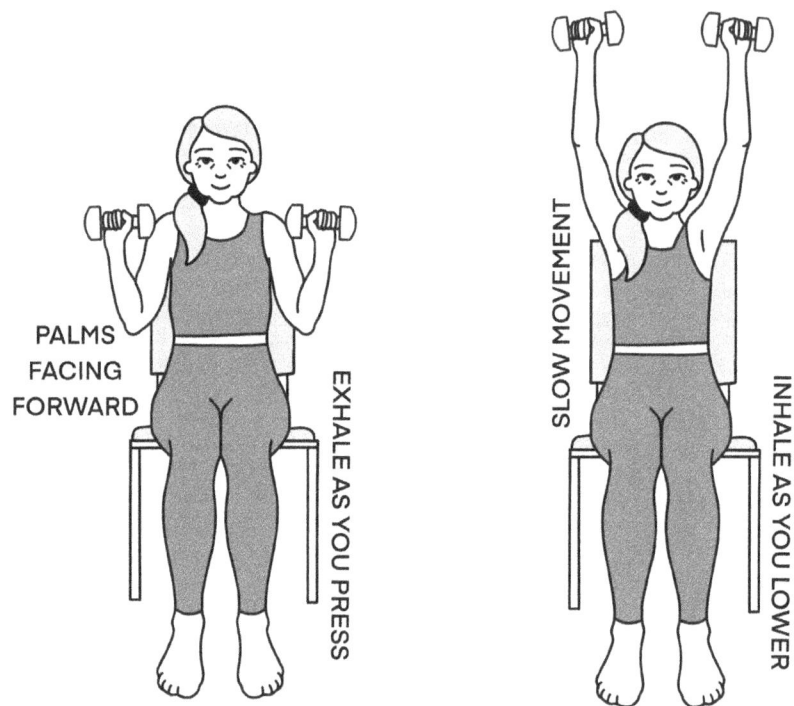

PALMS FACING FORWARD

EXHALE AS YOU PRESS

SLOW MOVEMENT

INHALE AS YOU LOWER

Focus: Shoulder muscles, mainly the anterior deltoid.

- Sit tall with your feet flat on the floor.

- Hold a light weight in each hand; begin with your elbows bent with the weights at shoulder level, and your palms facing forward.

- Slowly press the weights overhead, then lower the weights back to shoulder height.

- Perform a few sets of 10-15 repetitions.

Breathing: Exhale as you press the weights up and inhale as you lower them back down to shoulder level.

TRICEPS PULL DOWN

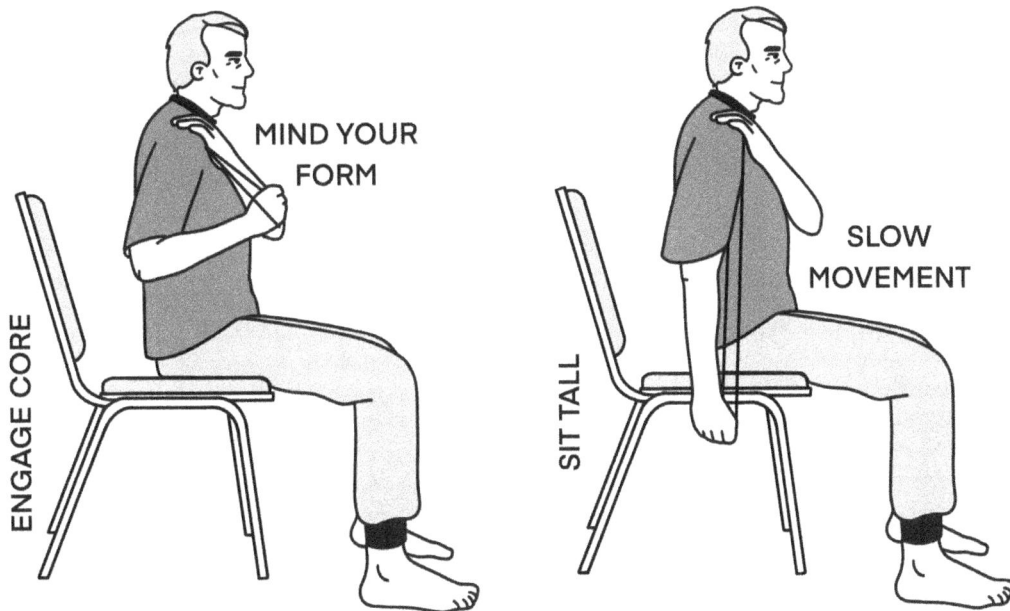

MIND YOUR FORM

ENGAGE CORE

SLOW MOVEMENT

SIT TALL

Focus: Strengthens the triceps.

- Sit tall with both feet on the floor.

- Place the end of an elastic band over your right shoulder and hold it down with your left hand.

- Hold the band with your right hand. (Your elbow should be bent.)

- Slowly straighten your forearm toward the floor while keeping the band anchored with your left hand, then bend your elbow again in a controlled manner.

- Perform a few sets of 10-15 repetitions.

Breathing: Exhale as you extend your elbow and inhale as your arm comes back up.

SHOULDER SHRUGS

Focus: Strengthens the neck and shoulder muscles, mainly the upper trapezius.

- Sit comfortably with your feet resting on the floor.

- Hold a light weight in each hand, and bring both arms out to the sides of your body at about a 30-degree angle.

- Shrug your shoulders toward your ears while keeping the angle in your arms, then relax the shoulders back down.

- Perform a few sets of 10-15 repetitions.

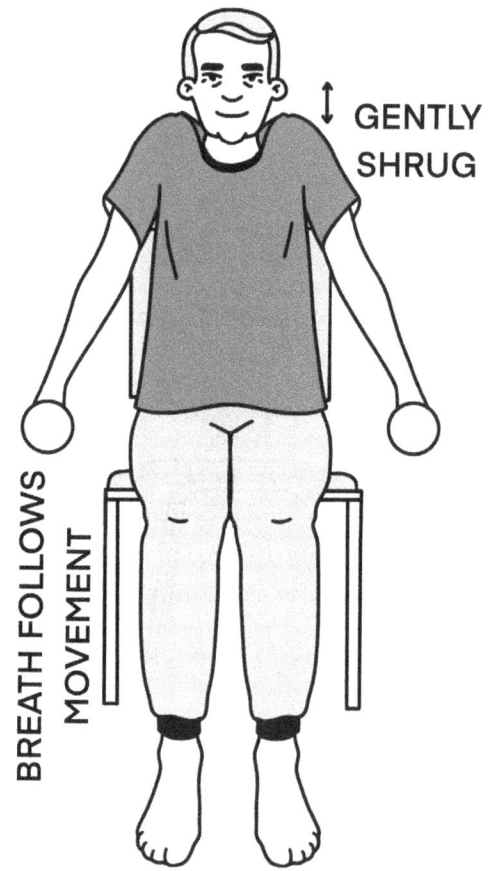

Breathing: Inhale as you shrug your shoulders and exhale as you relax them.

GENTLY SHRUG

BREATH FOLLOWS MOVEMENT

EXTERNAL ROTATION OF THE SHOULDER

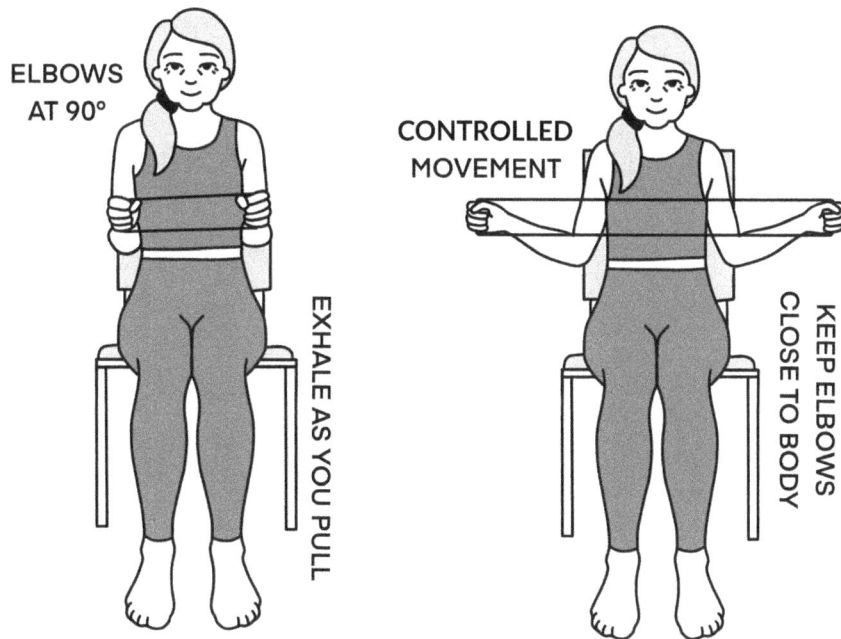

ELBOWS
AT 90°

EXHALE AS YOU PULL

CONTROLLED
MOVEMENT

KEEP ELBOWS
CLOSE TO BODY

Focus: Shoulder muscles, mainly the rotator cuff.

• Sit tall with both feet on the floor.

• Bend both elbows at 90 degrees and keep your arms tucked by your sides. Hold a resistance band with both hands. It should be forming a straight line right above your thighs.

• Slowly pull the band as if you want to tear it apart: rotate your forearms outward while keeping your elbows close to your body, then return to the starting position.

• Repeat for two sets of 10-15 repetitions.

Breathing: Exhale as you pull the band apart and inhale as you bring the arms back to midline.

EXERCISES FOR CHEST AND BACK

The chest and back muscles are essential for maintaining good posture and upper-body strength. The following exercises will help support these goals.

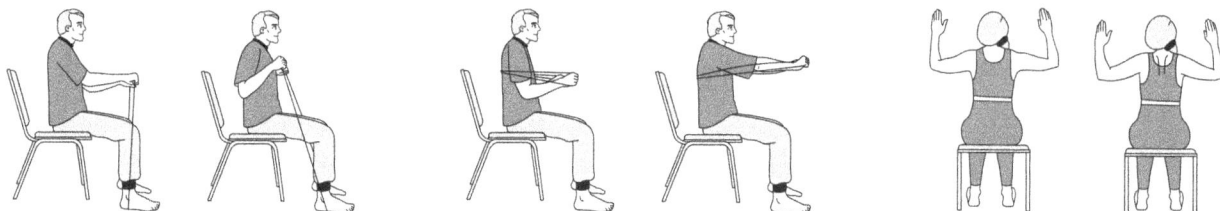

SEATED ROWS

UNDER TENSION

SIT TALL

FEET FLAT ON FLOOR

SQUEEZE YOUR SHOULDER BLADES

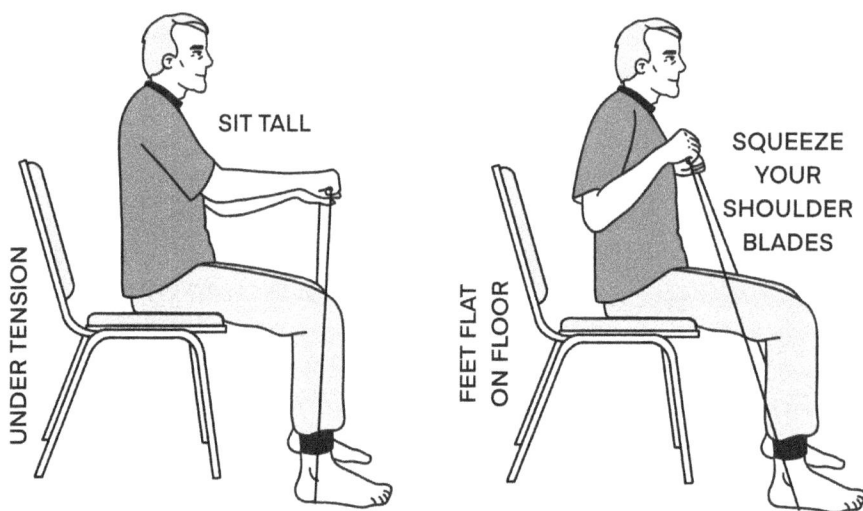

Focus: Strengthens the upper back, namely the latissimus dorsi and upper and middle trapezius.

Breathing: Exhale as you pull your elbows back and inhale as you release the tension on the band.

- Sit tall with your feet flat on the floor.

- Place a resistance band under both feet and hold one end in each hand so that there is some tension in the band. (Or, you can use a light weight in each hand.)

- Drive your elbows back while squeezing your shoulder blades together, then slowly return to the starting position.

- Perform a few sets of 10-15 repetitions.

CHEST PRESSES

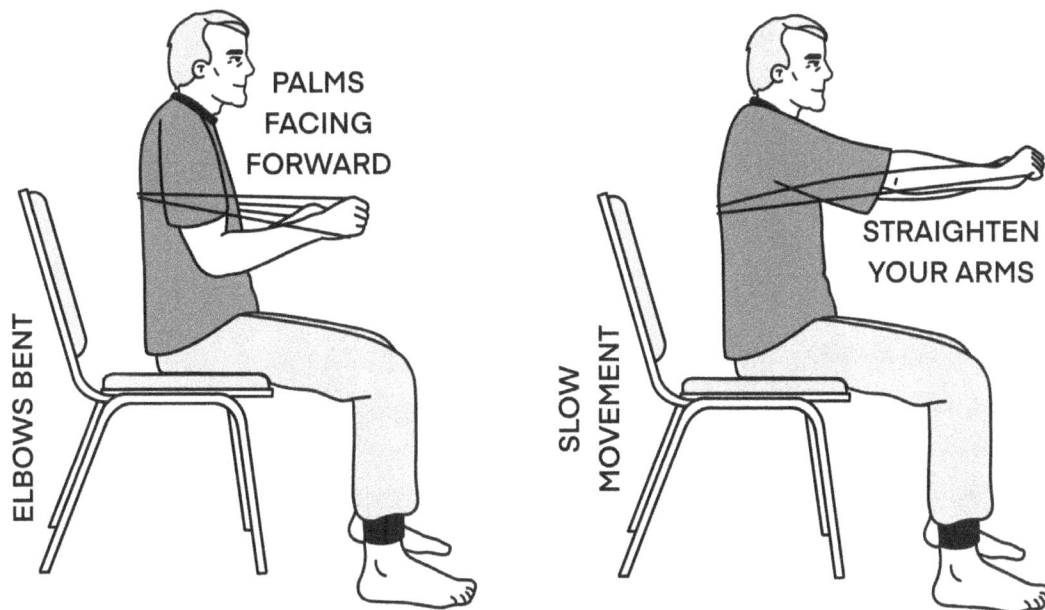

PALMS FACING FORWARD

ELBOWS BENT

STRAIGHTEN YOUR ARMS

SLOW MOVEMENT

Focus: Chest muscles, namely the pectoralis.

- Sit tall with your feet flat on the floor.

- Wrap a resistance band around your upper back, just below the shoulder blades.

- Hold one end of the band in each hand with your arms out to the side. Your elbows should be bent and your palms facing downward.

- Press your arms forward as you straighten them in front of you, then slowly return to the starting position.

- Perform a few sets of 10-15 repetitions.

Breathing: Exhale as you press your arms forward and inhale as you release the tension on the band.

SHOULDER BLADE SQUEEZES

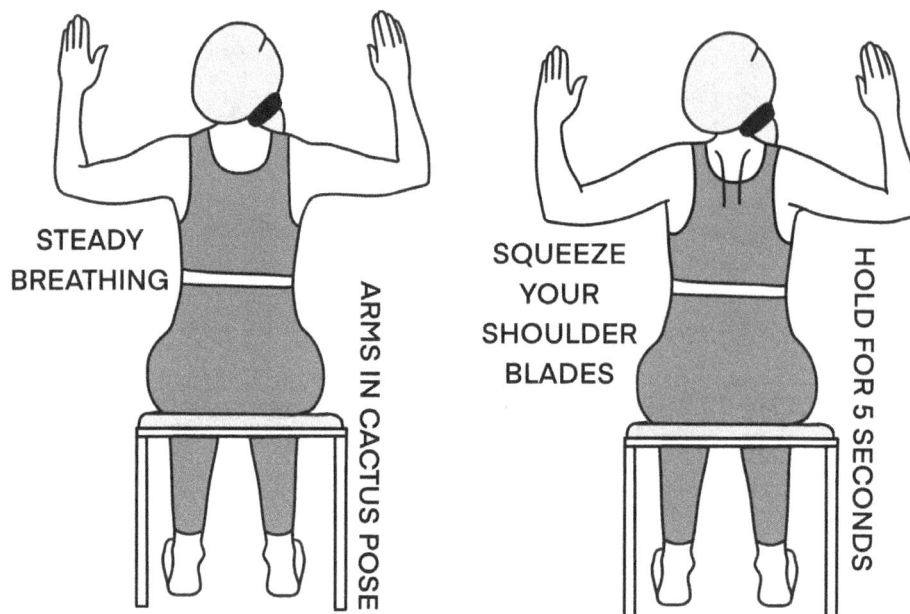

STEADY BREATHING

ARMS IN CACTUS POSE

SQUEEZE YOUR SHOULDER BLADES

HOLD FOR 5 SECONDS

Focus: Upper back muscles, mostly the rhomboids, middle trapezius, and lower trapezius.

- Sit with your feet flat on the floor.

- Take your arms into a cactus position. (Your shoulders and elbows should be at a 90-degree angle.)

- Slowly squeeze your shoulder blades together, as if you want to pinch something between them.

- Hold for a few seconds, then relax. Repeat ten times.

Breathing: Maintain steady breathing throughout the entire exercise.

All the above upper body strengthening exercises will be incorporated into the 4-Week Chair Exercise Program. They will help you maintain functional strength, improve posture, and maintain or improve your daily mobility. In the next chapter, we present the lower body strengthening exercises.

LOWER BODY STRENGTH EXERCISES

5

As we age, strengthening the lower body is crucial for maintaining and improving balance and range of motion. Increasing lower body strength will also allow you to preserve your independence. This means preserving the ability to carry out everyday activities like walking, getting up from a chair, and climbing stairs.

There are many ways to work on strengthening the lower body. Some examples include yoga, aquatic exercises, and strength training exercises with dumbbells, resistance bands, or machines. Research indicates that chair-based exercises are effective and should be encouraged as a simple, accessible way to maintain and build strength in older adults (Klempel et al., 2021). In this chapter, we'll explore a range of lower-body exercises that can be done while seated. These will target the main lower-body muscle groups such as your glutes, quads, hamstring, and calves.

We suggest using light weights or resistance bands for strengthening exercises. Remember that this is optional, and you are welcome to begin with active movements if that is more comfortable for you in the beginning.

EXERCISES FOR LEGS AND GLUTES

Preserving and building strength in the legs and glutes will help with balance, stability, and endurance in daily activities. The exercises presented below will allow you to work on the quadriceps, hamstrings, glutes, and hip flexors.

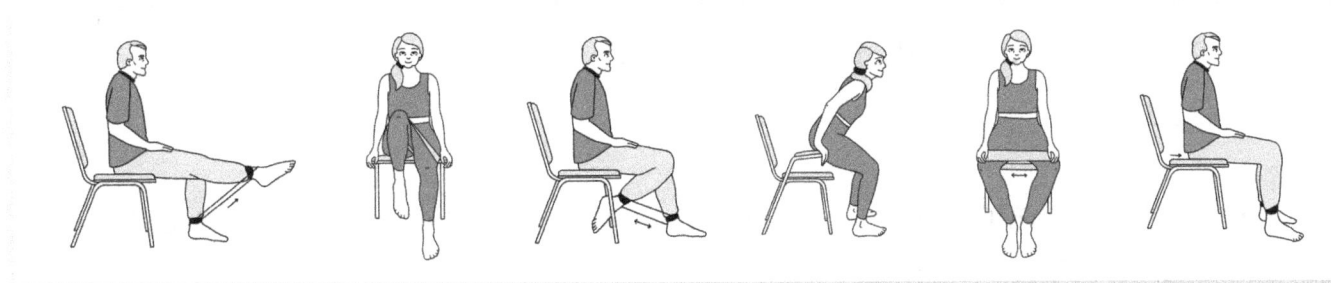

KNEE EXTENSIONS

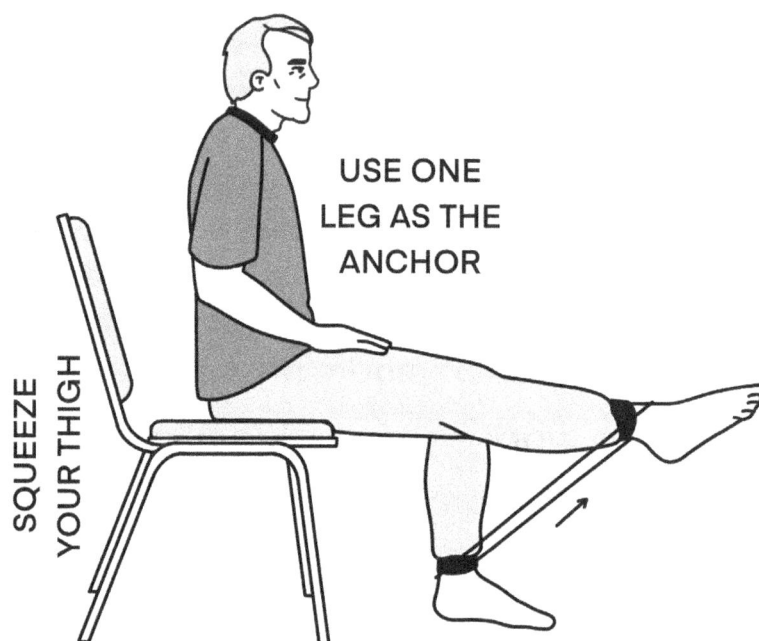

USE ONE
LEG AS THE
ANCHOR

SQUEEZE
YOUR THIGH

Focus: Strengthens the front of the thigh muscles called the quadriceps.

- Sit tall with your feet flat on the floor.

- Loop an elastic band around both ankles or use ankle weights for resistance.

- Extend one leg straight out in front of you, keeping the other foot flat on the floor. If you're using a resistance band, one of the legs stays still and anchors the band.

- Slowly lift one leg off the floor to try to straighten your knee. (The thigh should remain in contact with the chair.)

- Squeeze your thigh muscle (quadriceps) as if you want to move the kneecap toward you.

- Hold for a moment, then lower it back down.

- Repeat ten times on each leg.

Breathing: Exhale as you extend your leg and inhale as you release the leg down.

SEATED MARCHES

Focus: Strengthens the front of your hip and thigh muscles, namely the iliopsoas and quadriceps.

- Sit with your feet flat on the floor and your back straight.

- For resistance, place a band around both thighs (above the knee) or use ankle weights.

- Place your hands on the seat of the chair for support.

- Lift one knee toward your chest without letting your lower back round, then lower your knee and repeat with the opposite leg.

- Continue alternating the legs as if you are marching, ten times on each side.

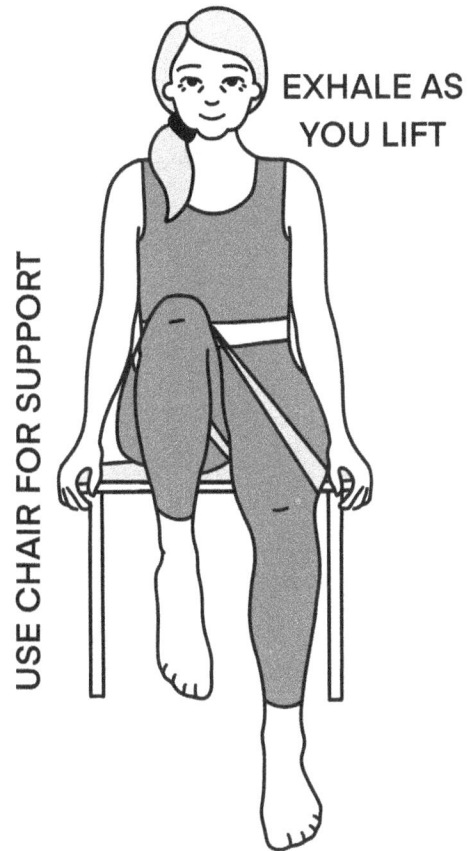

EXHALE AS YOU LIFT

USE CHAIR FOR SUPPORT

Breathing: Exhale as you lift your knee towards your chest and inhale as you release your leg down.

KNEE FLEXIONS

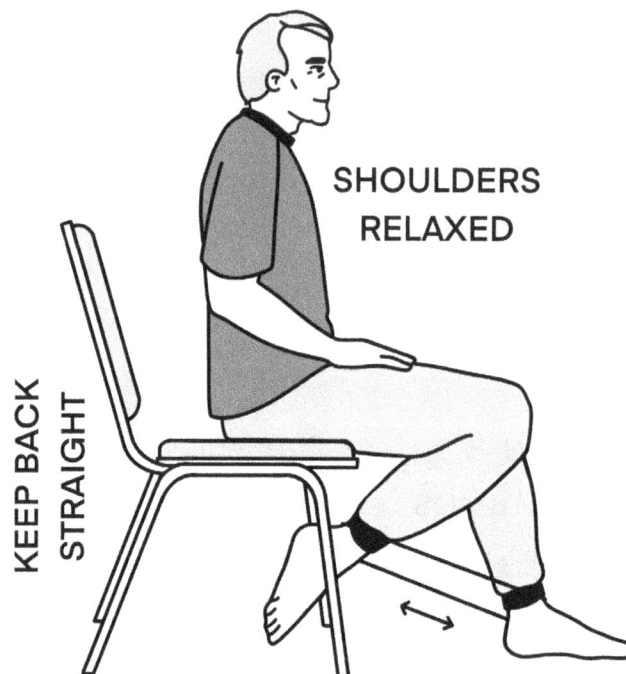

SHOULDERS
RELAXED

KEEP BACK
STRAIGHT

Focus: Strengthens the back of your thigh muscles, namely hamstrings.

- Sit on the edge of the chair with your feet flat on the floor.

- Loop a resistance band around your ankles.

- Extend one leg out in front of you to increase the tension on the band.

- Slowly bend the knee of the other leg to bring your heel toward the chair, then extend the leg back out. Repeat ten times on each side.

Breathing: Exhale as you bend your knee towards the chair and inhale as you extend the leg back out.

ASSISTED SQUATS

Focus: Strengthens the glutes and quadriceps.

- Sit near the edge of the chair with your feet flat on the floor, hip-width apart.

- Place your hands on the arms of the chair for support. Slowly stand up from the chair by pressing through your feet.

- Then, sit back down in a controlled manner. Avoid collapsing back onto the chair. Repeat ten times.

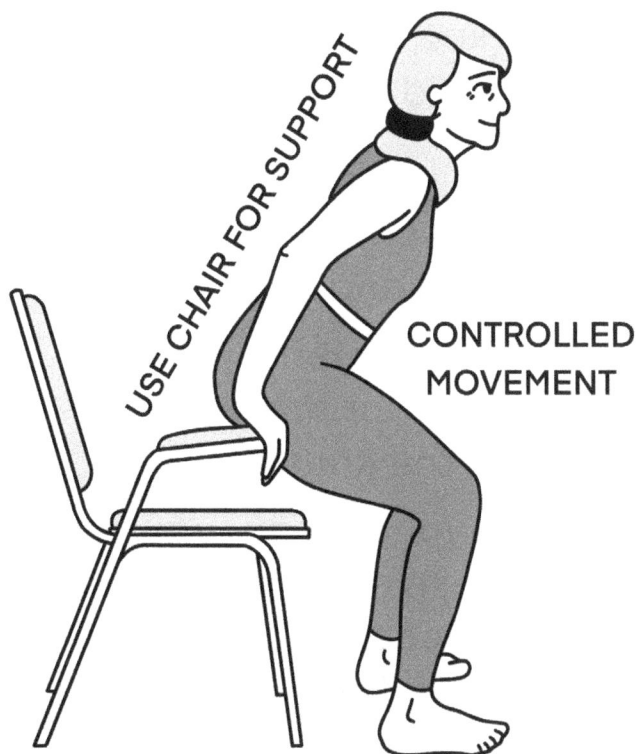

Breathing: Exhale as you push yourself up off the chair and inhale as you lower yourself back to sit on the chair.

USE CHAIR FOR SUPPORT

CONTROLLED MOVEMENT

CLAMS

Focus: Strengthens the side of the hips, namely the gluteus medius and minimus muscles.

- Sit tall in the chair with your feet flat on the floor. Keep your feet and thighs touching.

- Loop a resistance band around your thighs, right above the knees.

- Open your knees outward and push against the band; your feet should remain together. Then, slowly bring your knees back to the center.

- Repeat ten times.

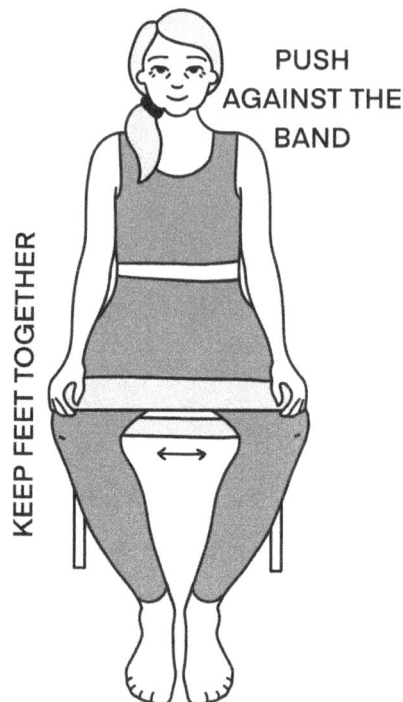

PUSH AGAINST THE BAND

KEEP FEET TOGETHER

Breathing: Exhale as you open your knees to push against the band and inhale as you bring your knees back together.

GLUTE SQUEEZE

Focus: Strengthens the back of the hips, namely the gluteus maximus muscle.

- Sit with your feet flat on the floor and your back straight.

- Squeeze your glutes as tightly as possible and hold for ten seconds, then release.

- Repeat ten times.

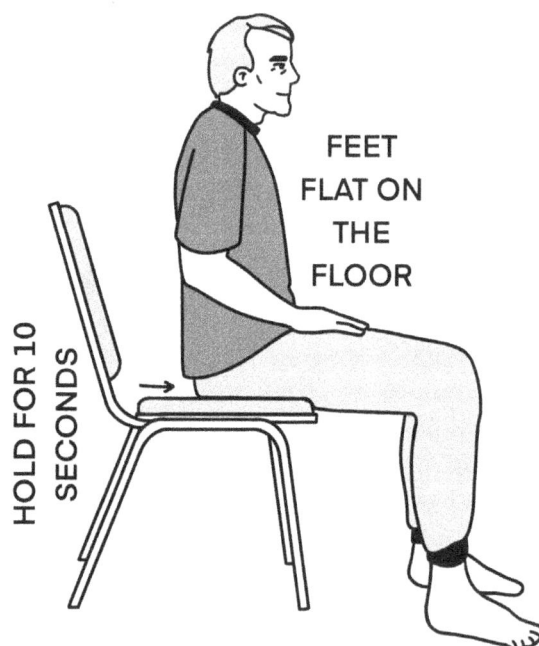

FEET FLAT ON THE FLOOR

HOLD FOR 10 SECONDS

Breathing: Maintain steady breathing throughout the entire exercise.

EXERCISES FOR ANKLES AND FEET

The following exercises will help strengthen the muscles in your lower legs, ankles, and feet, and consequently contribute to balance, stability and an overall steadier foundation for your daily activities.

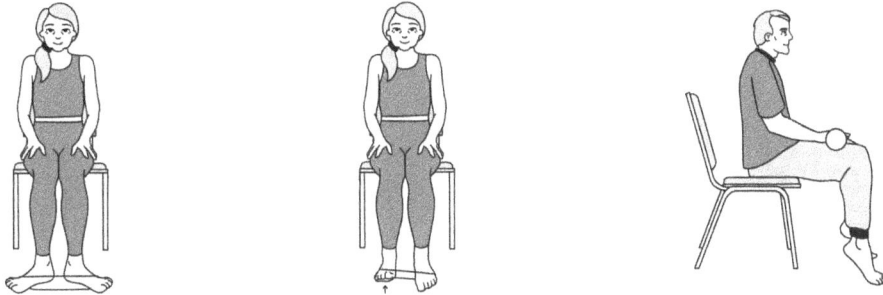

ANKLE EVERSIONS WITH A BAND

Focus: Strengthens the muscles around the ankle, especially the peroneals.

- Sit tall with your feet flat on the floor.

- Loop a resistance band around both feet.

- Keep your heels on the ground and slowly rotate your feet outward, pushing against the band.

- Hold the position for a moment, then slowly return to the starting position. Repeat ten times.

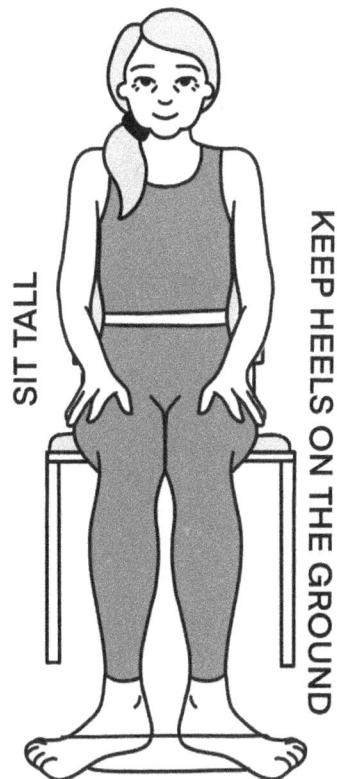

SIT TALL

KEEP HEELS ON THE GROUND

Breathing: Exhale as you push the feet against the band and inhale as bring the feet back towards midline.

TOE TAPS

Focus: Strengthens the muscles in the feet and shins, especially the tibialis anterior.

- Sit tall with your feet flat on the floor. Loop a resistance band around both feet.

- Lift your toes and one side of your foot off the ground while keeping your heel planted.

- The other foot should stay down to provide an anchor for the band.

- Tap your toes on the ground and lift them again. Repeat 15 times on each foot.

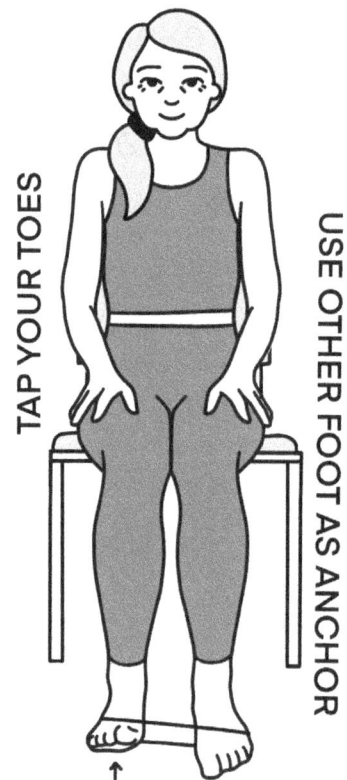

Breathing: Exhale as you lift your toes and foot off the ground and inhale as you lower them.

TAP YOUR TOES

USE OTHER FOOT AS ANCHOR

HEEL RAISES

Focus: Strengthens the calf muscles, namely the gastrocnemius and soleus.

- Sit with your feet flat on the floor. Place a dumbbell vertically on each thigh and hold it in place for the duration of the exercise.

- Lift your heels off the ground, rising onto the balls of your feet, then slowly lower your heels back down. Repeat fifteen times.

- If you want more, perform this exercise in a standing position. Place the chair against the wall and hold onto the backrest lightly for support. Come to the balls of your feet.

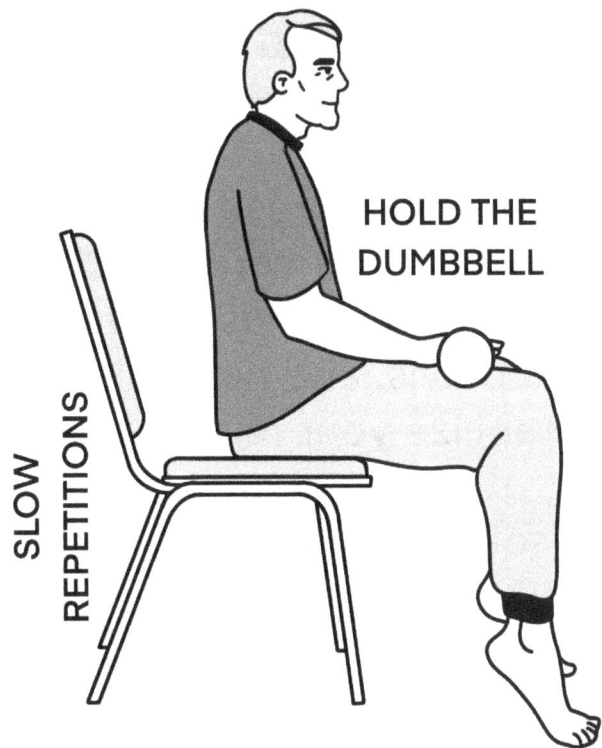

SLOW REPETITIONS

HOLD THE DUMBBELL

Breathing: Exhale as you lift your heels, and inhale as you lower them down.

These lower body strengthening exercises that were just presented will be added to the 4-Week Chair Exercise Program. They will help you improve or maintain your ability to walk, stand, and keep up with your daily activities. In the next chapter, we'll focus on core strengthening exercises you can perform with a chair. These are important in establishing a well-rounded strengthening routine.

CORE EXERCISES

6

The exercises presented in this chapter are designed to strengthen your core muscles. The core is a group of muscles located in your midsection. This includes your abdomen, lower back, pelvis, and hips. All together, these muscles engage to stabilize your midsection.

The following muscles are essential to core strength:

- Rectus abdominis (located at the front of the abdomen, the six-pack muscle).
- Internal and external obliques (located on the side of the abdomen).
- Transverse abdominis (located deep to the front of the abdominals).
- Diaphragm (breathing muscle).
- Erector spinae (located on either side of the spine).
- Multifidus (located deep to the erector spinae on either side of the spine).
- Glutes (located at the back of the hip).
- Pelvic floor (important for pelvic stability and continence).

Essentially, we can see these muscles as a natural corset to stabilize the midsection. They form a box with some located at the front, back, sides, top, and bottom of the midsection. Strengthening the core has been shown to improve balance and weight distribution in the elderly. It is also recommended as part of an effective strategy to prevent falls (Kang, 2015).

EXERCISES FOR CORE STRENGTH

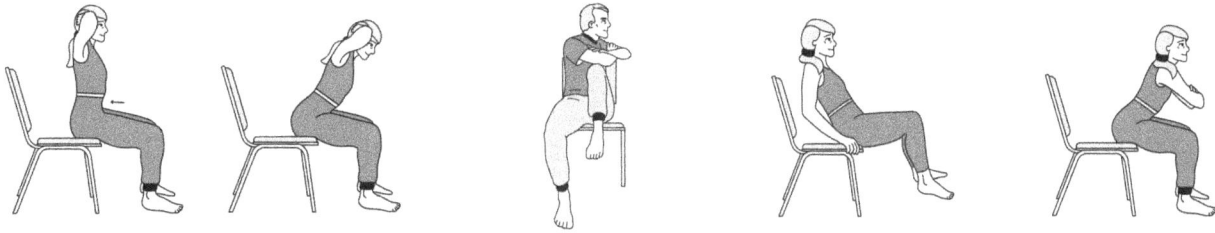

ABDOMINAL CRUNCHES

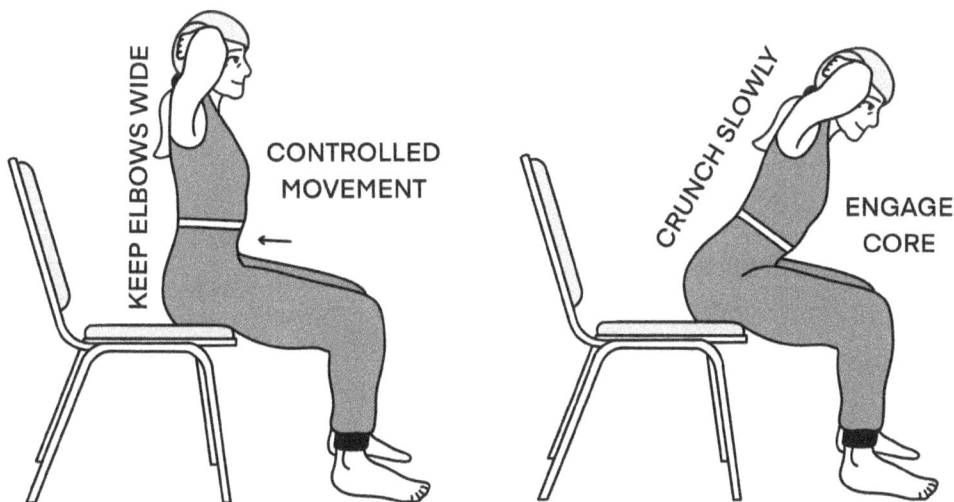

Focus: Strengthens the front of the abdomen, namely the rectus abdominis.

- Sit tall close to the edge of the chair with your feet flat on the floor.
- Place your hands behind your head and keep your elbows wide.
- Pull your belly button towards your spine as you crunch forward slowly, then return to the starting position as you release the tension in your abdomen. Repeat 10-15 times.

Breathing: Exhale as you pull your belly button in and crunch. Inhale as you return to the starting position with a straight spine.

OBLIQUE TWISTS

Focus: Engages the side of the abdomen, namely the internal and external obliques.

- Sit tall close to the edge of the chair with your feet flat on the floor.

- Cross your arms over your chest.

- Keep your back straight and twist your torso to the right, as you lift your right knee. Try to touch your left elbow to your right knee, then return to the center and repeat to the left.

- Repeat ten times on each side.

KEEP BACK STRAIGHT

EXHALE ON TWIST

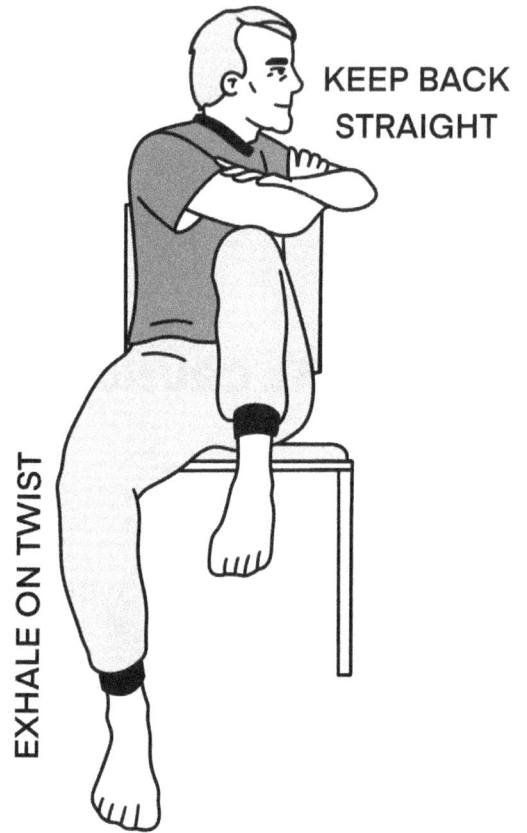

Breathing: Exhale as you twist to one side and inhale as you return to the center.

LEG TUCKS

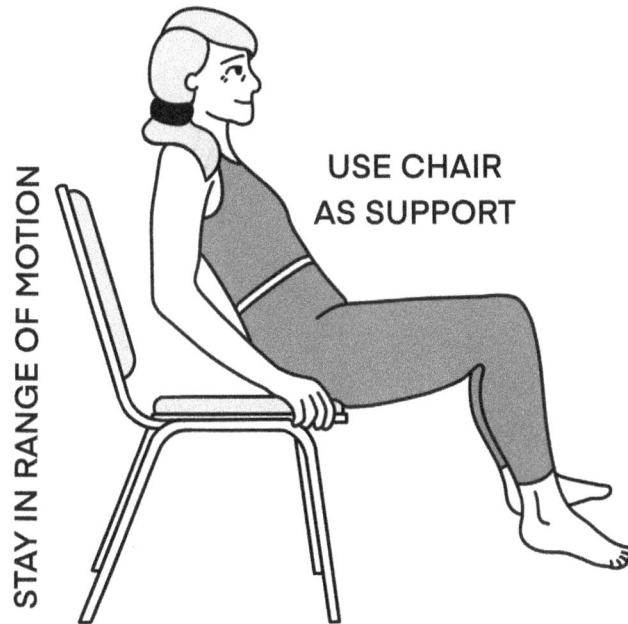

STAY IN RANGE OF MOTION

USE CHAIR AS SUPPORT

Focus: Strengthens the lower abdominals and hip flexors, promoting better lower body control.

- Sit tall close to the edge of the chair and place your hands on the sides of the seat for support.

- Lean back slightly while keeping your back straight, while extending your legs out in front of you. Let them hover over the floor; then bring your legs back to the initial position as you straighten your spine.

- Repeat 10-15 times.

Breathing: Inhale as you lean back and extend your legs out. Exhale as you pull your legs back in and straighten your spine.

BACK EXTENSIONS

Focus: Targets the posterior aspect of the core, namely the erector spinae and multifidus.

- Sit tall with your feet flat on the floor hip-distance apart.

- Cross your arms over your chest and keep your shoulders relaxed.

- Hinge at your hips and lean forward while keeping your back straight, then slowly return to an upright position by engaging your back muscles.

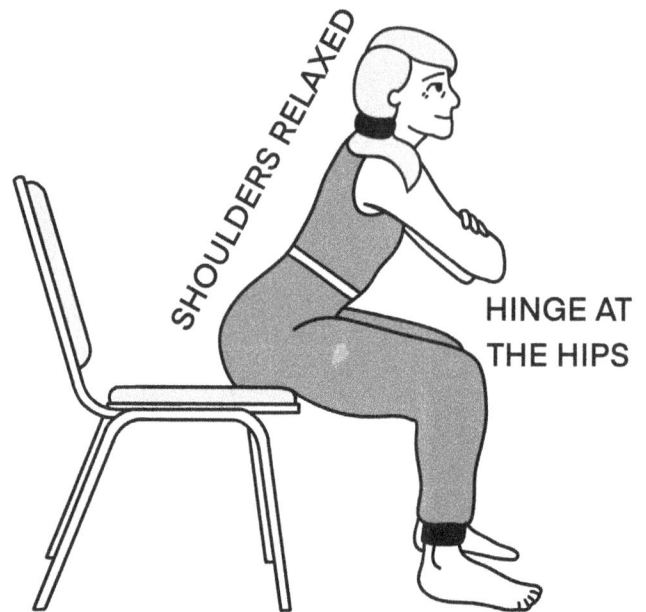

- Repeat 10-15 times.

SHOULDERS RELAXED

HINGE AT THE HIPS

Breathing: Inhale as you hinge forward and exhale as you lift yourself back up to the starting position.

These core exercises are an effective way to improve your stability and confidence in everyday activities. Because they are performed in a seated position, they may also reduce the stress on your lower back. Be sure to pay attention to any pain or discomfort you may be feeling and respect your current limitations.

In the next chapter, we dive into chair flexibility exercises that will help you move more freely in your everyday life.

FLEXIBILITY EXERCISES

7

Reduced flexibility in older adults can lead to many issues like postural imbalance, restricted movement, and changes in walking characteristics (like speed, stride length, walking frequency, and joint range of motion). These limitations can hinder daily activities and eventually lower quality of life. Also, a decreased range of motion increases the risk of falling (La Greca et al., 2022).

The American College of Sports Medicine (ACSM) defines flexibility as the ability to move through a full joint range of motion. Stretching, for example, is one way to improve flexibility. It's important to mention that other methods of training, such as strength training in a full range of motion, have also been shown to improve flexibility (Afonso et al., 2021). The stretching exercises in this chapter will focus on improving flexibility in key muscle groups.

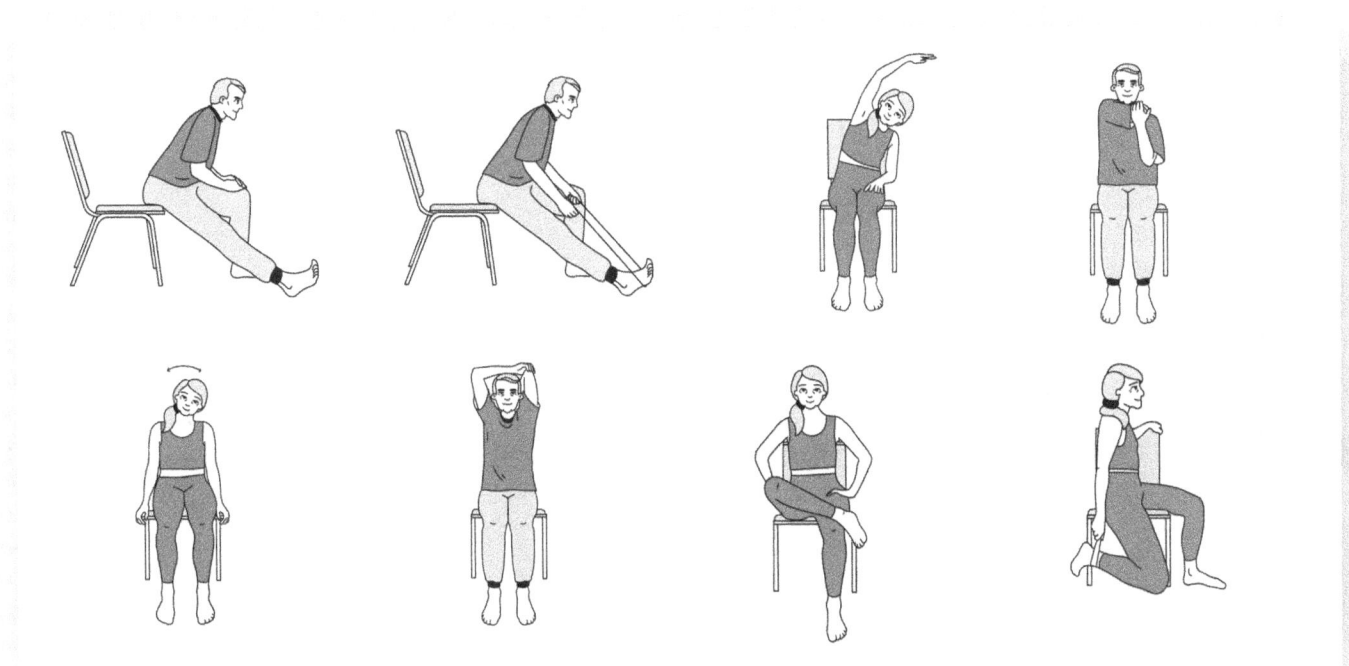

HAMSTRING STRETCH

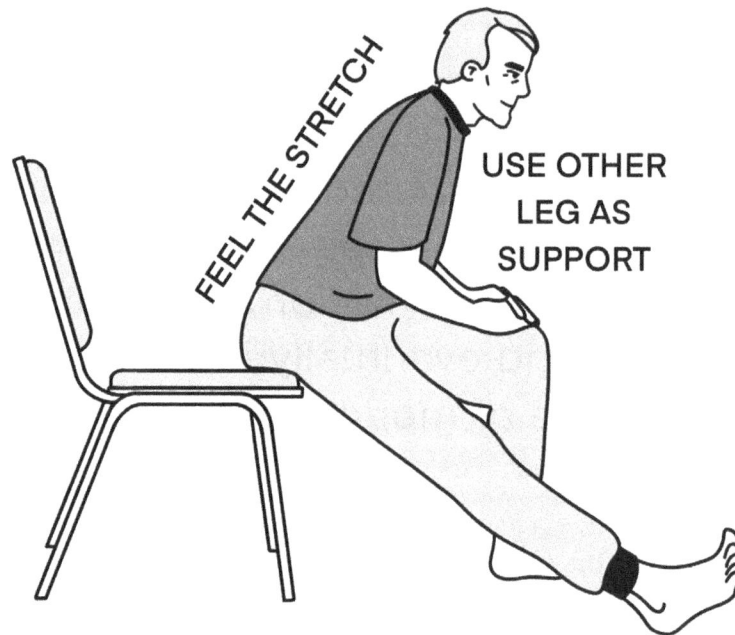

FEEL THE STRETCH

USE OTHER
LEG AS
SUPPORT

Focus: Stretches the back of the hip and thigh.

- Sit at the edge of the chair with a tall spine.

- Extend one leg straight in front of you and maintain your heel on the floor; place your hands on the other thigh for support.

- Hinge slowly forward from your hips; reach your torso toward your toes while keeping your back straight.

- Hold for 20-30 seconds, then switch legs.

- Repeat a few times on each side.

Breathing: Maintain steady breathing throughout the entire stretch.

CALF STRETCH

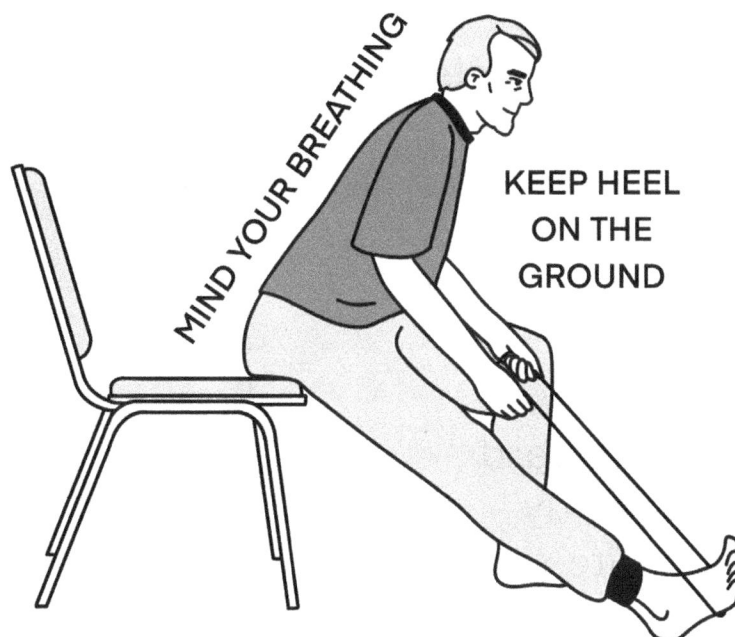

MIND YOUR BREATHING

KEEP HEEL
ON THE
GROUND

Focus: Stretches the calf muscles, namely the gastrocnemius and soleus.

- Sit at the edge of the chair with a tall spine.

- Extend one leg in front of you and keep your heel on the floor.

- Place a yoga strap around the ball of your foot and hold the ends with each hand.

- Gently pull your toes toward you while keeping your heel on the ground. Hold for 20-30 seconds, then switch legs.

- Repeat a few times on each side.

Breathing: Maintain steady breathing throughout the entire stretch.

OVERHEAD REACHES

Focus: Stretches the side of the torso and shoulder muscles, namely the latissimus dorsi, deltoids, obliques, and intercostal muscles.

- Sit tall with your feet flat on the floor.

- Raise one arm overhead and reach gently toward the ceiling and slightly over to the opposite side.

- You should feel a stretch along your side and through your shoulder where the arm is lifted. Hold for 20-30 seconds, then switch arms.

- Repeat a few times on each side.

KEEP FEET ON FLOOR

FEEL THE STRETCH

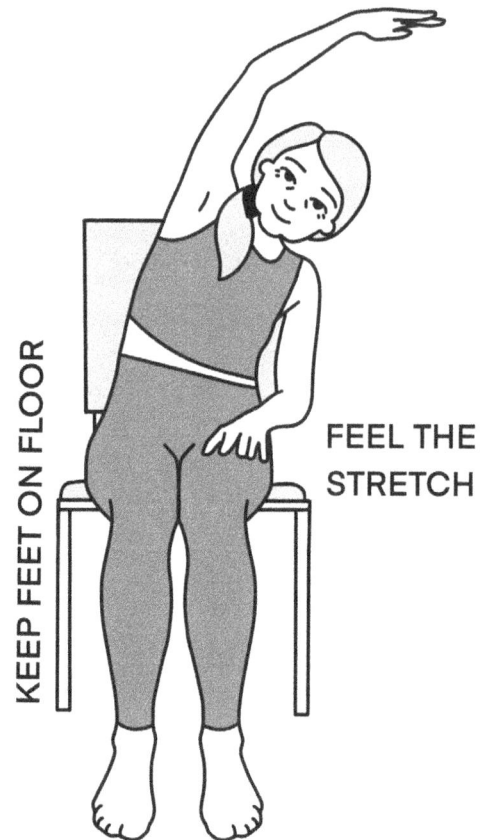

Breathing: Maintain steady breathing throughout the entire stretch.

CROSS-BODY ARM STRETCH

Focus: Stretches the back of the shoulder and upper back muscles, namely the posterior deltoid, middle trapezius, and rhomboids.

- Sit tall with your feet flat on the floor.

- Bring one arm across your body at chest height.

- Pull it gently toward your chest by applying pressure at the back of your arm with the opposite hand.

- You should feel a stretch at the back of your shoulder or mid-back. Go easy if you feel pinching at the front of your shoulder. Hold for 20-30 seconds, then switch arms.

- Repeat a few times on each side.

GENTLY APPLY PRESSURE

FEEL THE STRETCH

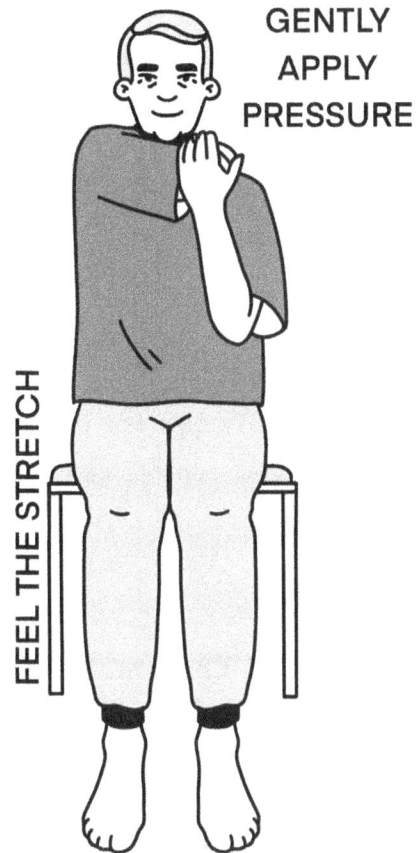

Breathing: Maintain steady breathing throughout the entire stretch.

UPPER TRAP STRETCH

Focus: Stretches the side of the neck and upper shoulder, namely the upper trapezius muscle.

- Sit tall with both feet on the floor.

- Place one hand on the side of the chair gripping the under part of the seat to stabilize your shoulder.

- Tilt your head to the opposite side. You should feel the stretch along the side of your neck and your upper shoulder. If you want more, use your other hand to gently pull on your head. Hold for thirty seconds, then switch sides.

- Repeat a few times on each side.

FEEL THE STRETCH

USE CHAIR FOR SUPPORT

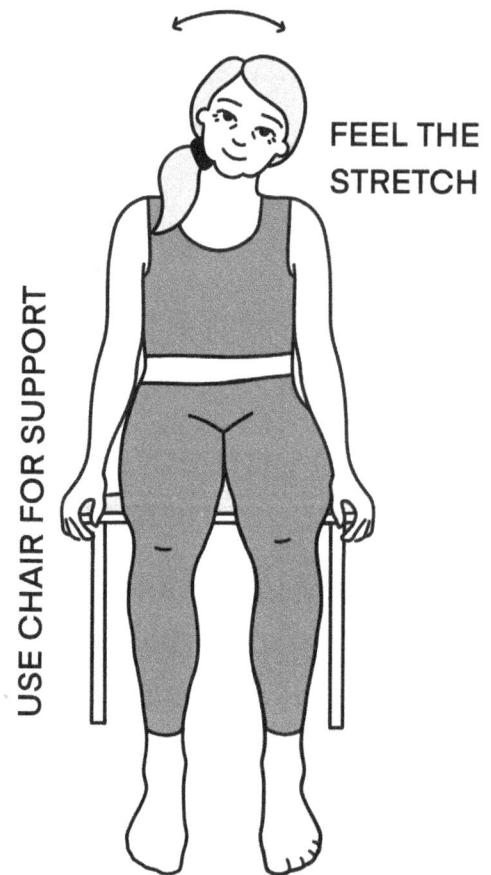

Breathing: Maintain steady breathing throughout the entire stretch.

TRICEPS STRETCH

Focus: Stretches the back of the upper arm and shoulder, namely the triceps muscle.

- Sit tall with both feet on the floor.

- Raise one arm overhead and bend the elbow; let your hand fall behind your back. With the opposite hand, gently press on the raised elbow.

- Hold for thirty seconds, then switch arms.

- Repeat a few times on each side.

Breathing: Maintain steady breathing throughout the entire stretch.

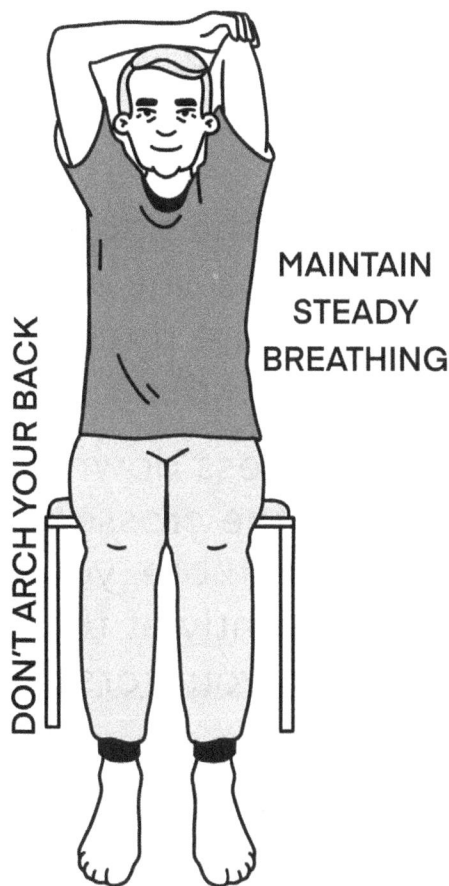

DON'T ARCH YOUR BACK

MAINTAIN STEADY BREATHING

FIGURE-4 STRETCH

Focus: Stretches the back and outer hip, namely the glute muscles.

- Sit tall at the edge of the chair. Cross one ankle over the opposite thigh, just above the knee.

- Gently press down on the knee of the crossed leg. If you want more, you can hinge slightly at the hips and lean your torso forward.

- Hold for thirty seconds, then switch legs.

- Repeat a few times on each side.

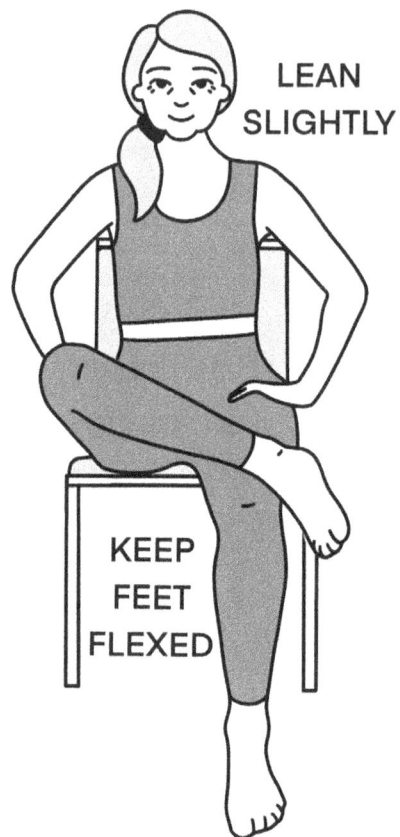

Breathing: Maintain steady breathing throughout the entire stretch.

LEAN SLIGHTLY

KEEP FEET FLEXED

QUAD STRETCH

Focus: Stretches the front of the hip and thigh, namely the quadriceps muscle.

- Sit sideways in the chair with one leg hanging off the side.

- Hold onto the back of the chair for support.

- Place a yoga strap around the front of the ankle of the leg hanging off to the side.

- Slowly begin to bend your knee to stretch the front of the thigh by pulling back with the towel or strap. Hold for thirty seconds, then switch sides.

- Repeat a few times on each side.

SIT TALL

HOLD ONTO
THE CHAIR

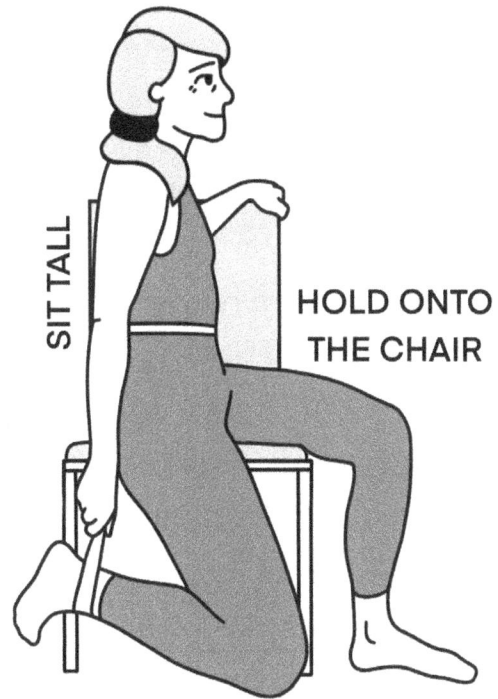

Breathing: Maintain steady breathing throughout the entire stretch.

The stretches presented in this chapter will create more ease of movement and increase comfort in daily activities. Incorporating flexibility work regularly supports overall wellness and should be part of any comprehensive workout routine.

In the next chapter, we'll focus on balance and stability exercises that can be performed on a chair.

BALANCE AND STABILITY EXERCISES

8

Working on core strength, stability, and balance can be extremely beneficial for maintaining an active lifestyle as you age. Having optimal balance and stability is crucial for preventing falls and maintaining confidence and independence in daily activities. Studies show that as many as 30% of adults over the age of 65 will experience problems with balance or dizziness, which can lead to falls and injuries (Wang et al., 2024). Balance is defined as the ability to maintain our center of gravity over our base of support. There are two types of balance: **Static balance** occurs when you maintain stability while still. **Dynamic balance** happens when you maintain stability during movement (O'Sullivan et al., 2014, p.187).

Balance is complex and is influenced by multiple systems:

Visual: Helps us position our body appropriately and maintain balance through our eyes.

Proprioceptive: Provides information to our body obtained from receptors present in our skin, tendons, joints, and muscles.

Vestibular: This system includes our inner ear and vestibular centers in our brain. It helps us keep our balance by analyzing our head movements in our surrounding space.

Balance is often used interchangeably with other terms like postural stability and postural control. For the sake of this book, we will be using the terms balance and stability interchangeably. The following exercises are designed to improve your postural stability. A chair is used either to support the entire body while sitting or as assistance while challenging the balance in standing. As you exercise, remember to maintain steady breathing throughout all of the exercises.

BALANCE EXERCISES

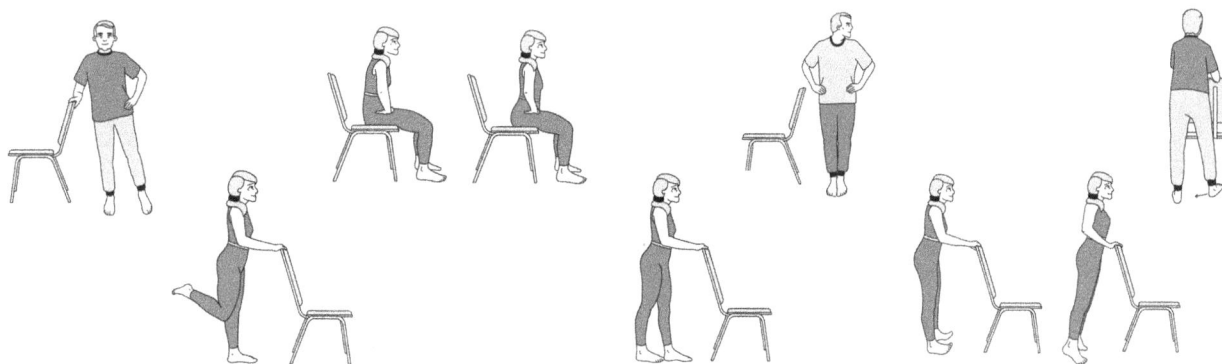

WEIGHT SHIFTS

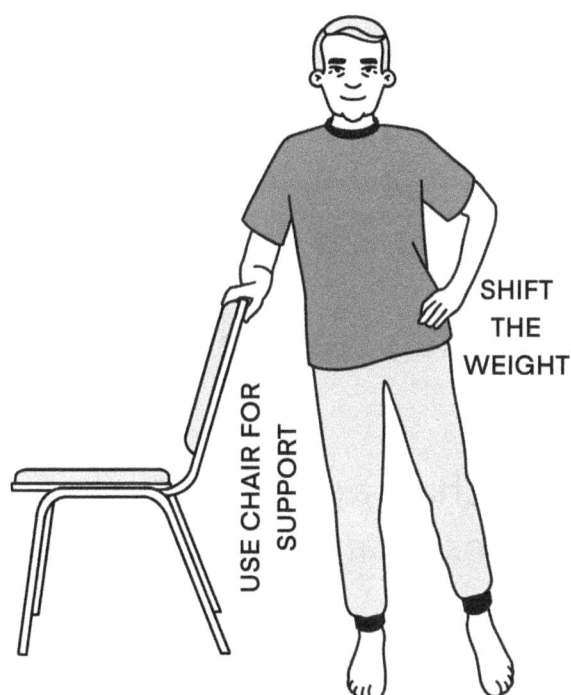

USE CHAIR FOR SUPPORT

SHIFT THE WEIGHT

Focus: Improves awareness of the hips and ankles as well as builds confidence in offloading one limb.

• Securely prop your chair against a wall, stand behind it and hold onto the backrest for support.

• Shift your weight slowly to one foot, and lift the opposite foot off the ground.

• Repeat ten times on each side while using controlled movements and engaging your core for stability.

ONE-LEGGED STANCE

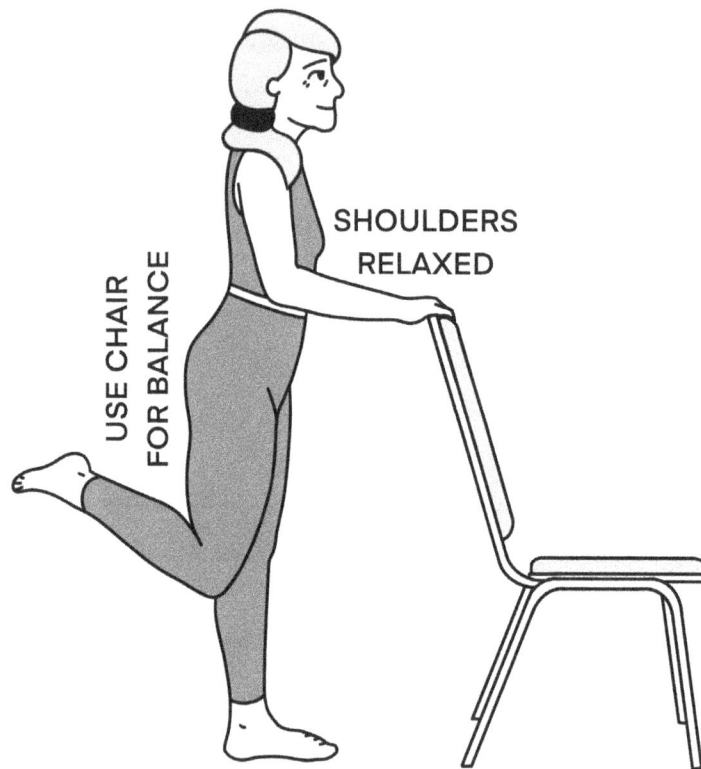

SHOULDERS RELAXED

USE CHAIR FOR BALANCE

Focus: Improves single-leg static balance and works on hip and ankle stability.

- Securely prop your chair against a wall, stand behind it and hold onto the backrest for support. Place your feet hip-distance apart.

- Keep your back straight and your shoulders relaxed. Bend one knee and lift your foot behind you, so that you are only standing on one leg.

- Maintain your balance with the weight evenly distributed on the four corners of your foot. Do not grip your toes. Let go of the chair if possible.

- Hold the position for 15-20 seconds, then release. Repeat a few times on each side.

PELVIC TILTS

SHOULDERS RELAXED

SHIFT YOUR WEIGHT

HANDS ON HIPS

KEEP BACK STRAIGHT

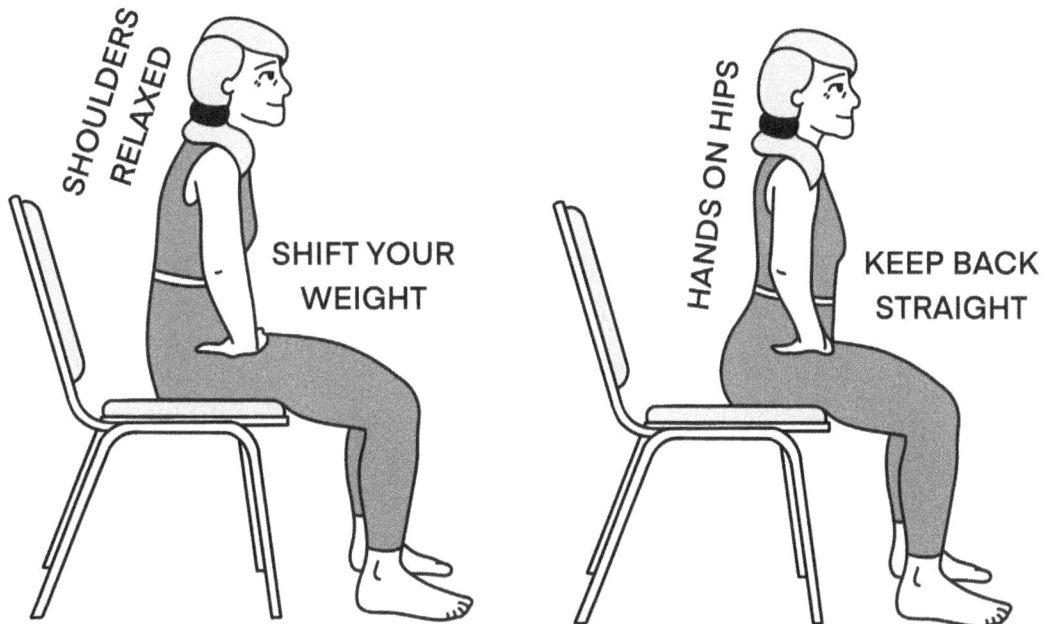

Focus: Improves core stability and works on lower back and pelvis range of motion.

- Sit in a chair with an upright posture and relaxed shoulders. Keep your back straight; do not rest against the backrest.

- Place your feet hip-distance apart, and your hands on your hips.

- Shift your weight slightly forward and allow your lower back to gently arch (anterior tilt), then return to a neutral position.

- Shift your weight backward and allow your lower back to gently round (posterior tilt).

- Repeat ten times.

TANDEM STANCE

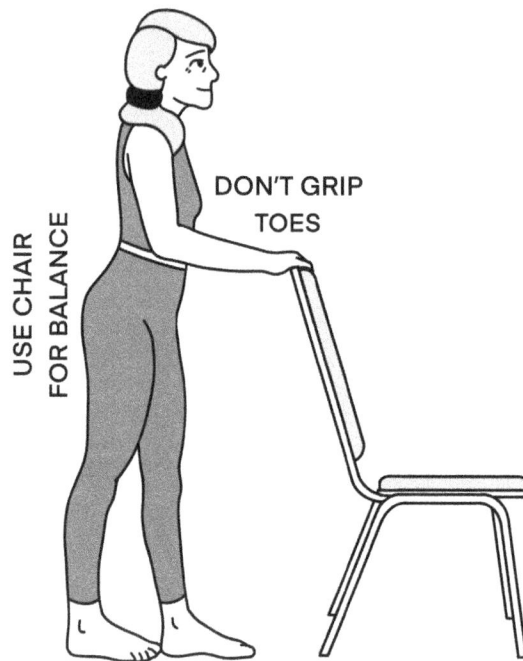

USE CHAIR FOR BALANCE

DON'T GRIP TOES

Focus: Improves static balance with a narrower base of support and works on ankle stability.

- Securely prop your chair against a wall, stand behind it and hold onto the backrest for support. Place your feet in a tandem stance with the heel of one foot directly in front of the toes of the other foot.

- Keep your back straight and your shoulders relaxed. Maintain your balance with an equal amount of weight on both feet. Do not grip your toes.

- Hold the position for thirty seconds, then release and repeat a few times on each side.

NARROW STANCE WITH NECK ROTATION

Focus: Improves dynamic balance by incorporating head and neck movement, which mimics real-world challenges.

- Securely prop your chair against a wall, stand behind it and hold onto the backrest for support. Place your feet side by side so they are touching each other.

- Keep your back straight and your shoulders relaxed. Let go of the chair and place your hands on your hips.

- Maintain your balance with an equal amount of weight on both feet. Do not grip your toes.

- Turn your head to look to the left, come back through the center, and turn your head to the right. Repeat ten times.

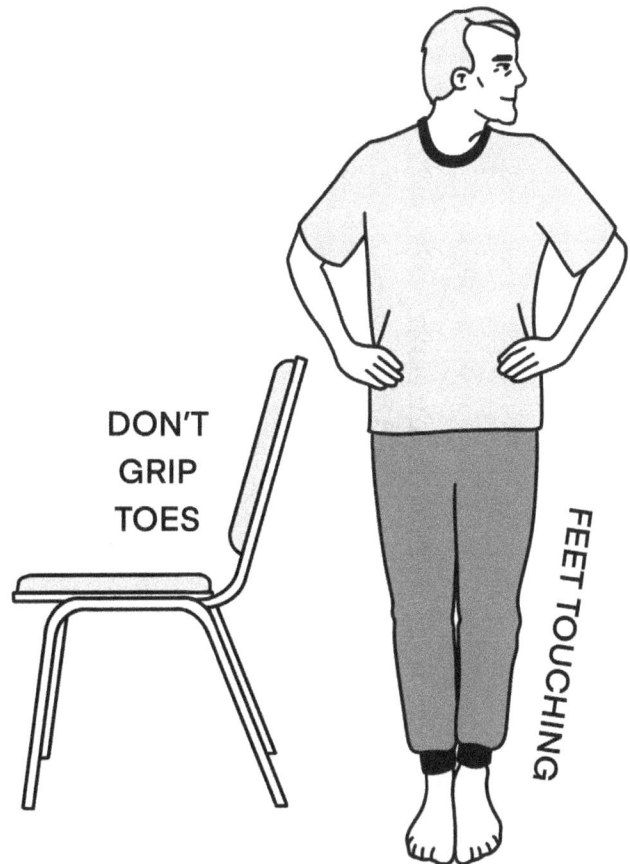

DON'T GRIP TOES

FEET TOUCHING

HEEL-TO-TOE ROCKING

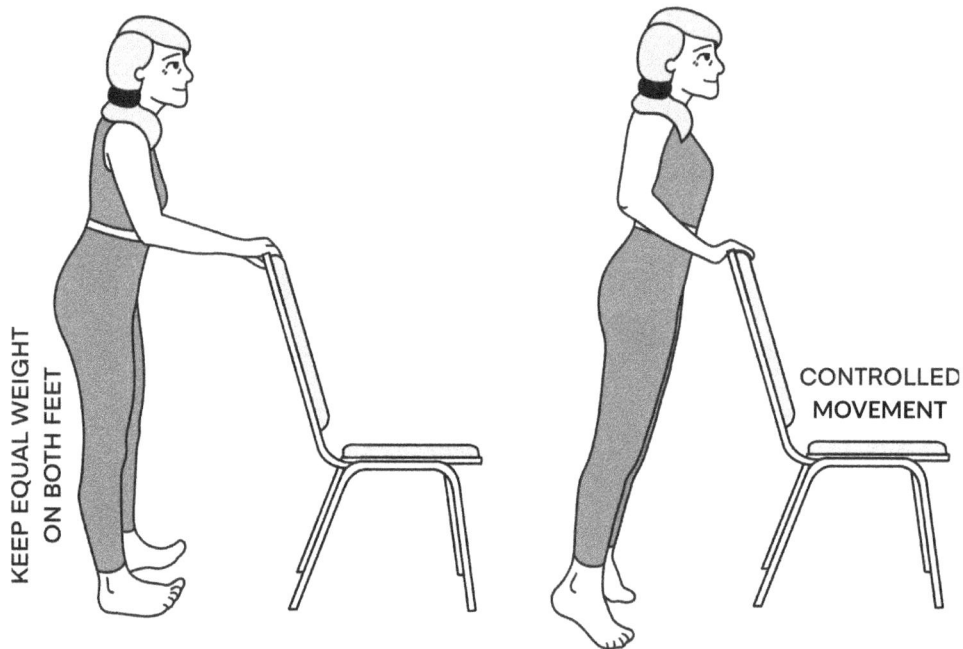

KEEP EQUAL WEIGHT ON BOTH FEET

CONTROLLED MOVEMENT

Focus: Improves dynamic balance, as well as ankle strength and mobility.

- Securely prop your chair against a wall, stand behind it and hold onto the backrest for support. Place your feet hip-distance apart with equal weight on both feet.

- Keep your back straight and your shoulders relaxed. Slowly rock backward to shift your weight in your heels so your toes lift off the floor.

- Then rock forward to shift the weight to the balls of your feet so your heels lift off the floor. Rock back and forth, controlling both directions of the movement.

- Repeat ten times.

STANDING SIDESTEP

Focus: Improves dynamic lateral balance and strengthens the hip muscles.

- Securely prop your chair against a wall, stand behind it and hold onto the backrest for support. Place your feet hip-distance apart with equal weight on both feet.

- Keep your back straight and your shoulders relaxed. Step sideways with your right foot, bringing the left foot to meet it.

- Then, reverse the motion by stepping out with your left foot and bringing the right foot to meet it. Repeat ten times in each direction.

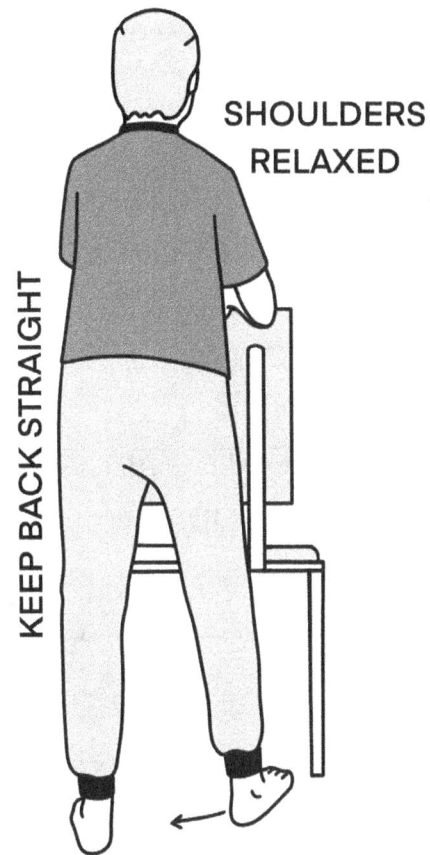

SHOULDERS RELAXED

KEEP BACK STRAIGHT

By incorporating these movements into your regular exercise routine, not only will your balance improve, but you will feel more confident in your daily activities. In the next chapter, we focus on chair-based exercises to improve your cardiovascular health.

LOW IMPACT AEROBIC EXERCISES

9

There are normal changes that occur with aging within the cardiovascular system (heart and blood vessels). These changes can raise the risk of heart disease and related health issues, which can significantly impact activity and quality of life (National Institute on Aging, 2024). Luckily, there are ways to prevent and reduce the risk of cardiovascular disease. Exercise is one piece of the puzzle. The National Institute on Aging recommends 150 minutes of moderate-intensity cardiovascular exercise per week.

The exercises presented in this chapter are a good way to increase your cardio minutes. However, we recommend completing the recommended time with other activities like walking, swimming, and dancing.

When you begin, if you can't reach 150 minutes of cardiovascular exercise each week, just aim to build up to it gradually. A good way to build up is to spread your cardio activities throughout the day. Research shows that brief sessions of exercise (such as ten minutes of aerobic exercise, three times per day) can have similar effects to longer workouts on cardiovascular health (Magutah et al., 2020).

Other factors to look out for to take care of your heart health include:

- Avoid smoking.
- Limit your alcohol intake.
- Eat a healthy diet, including food high in protein and fiber, but low in saturated fat, sugar, and salt.
- Maintain a healthy weight.

- Learn to manage stress levels.

- Practice good sleep hygiene.

- Monitor your blood pressure, blood glucose (sugar) levels, and cholesterol levels with routine checkups.

The chair-based exercises below are designed to provide a safe yet effective workout to get your heart rate up safely, all while making it accessible with a chair. Maintain steady breathing throughout all of the exercises.

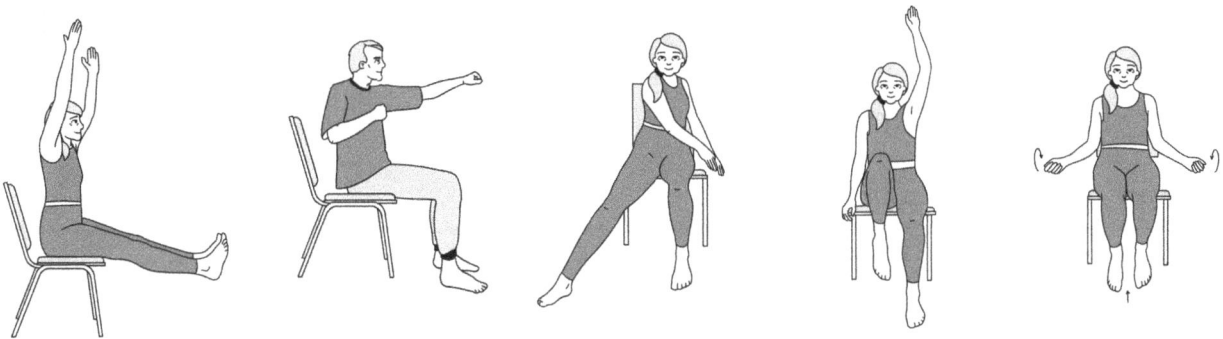

SEATED JUMPING JACKS

Focus: Elevates the heart rate and improves coordination.

- Sit tall with your feet flat on the floor and your arms resting at your sides.

- Lift both arms overhead while extending your legs. Return to the starting position and repeat.

- Perform for 30 seconds.

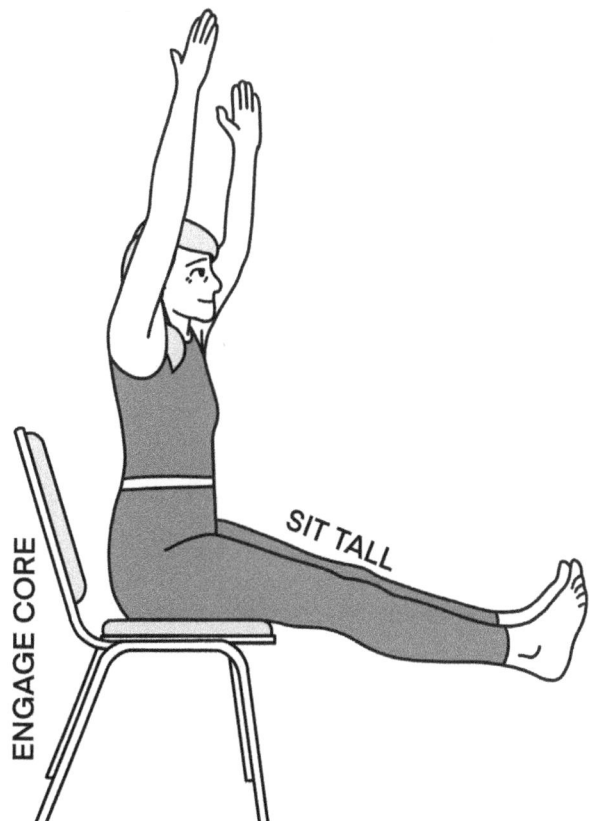

ENGAGE CORE

SIT TALL

SEATED PUNCHES

Focus: Increases cardiovascular endurance, improves arm strength, and engages the core.

- Sit tall with your feet flat on the floor. Raise your fists near your shoulders.

- Punch one arm forward while rotating slightly through the torso on that side.

- Alternate your arms in a steady motion. Pick up the speed as you get comfortable with the movement.

- Perform for 30 seconds.

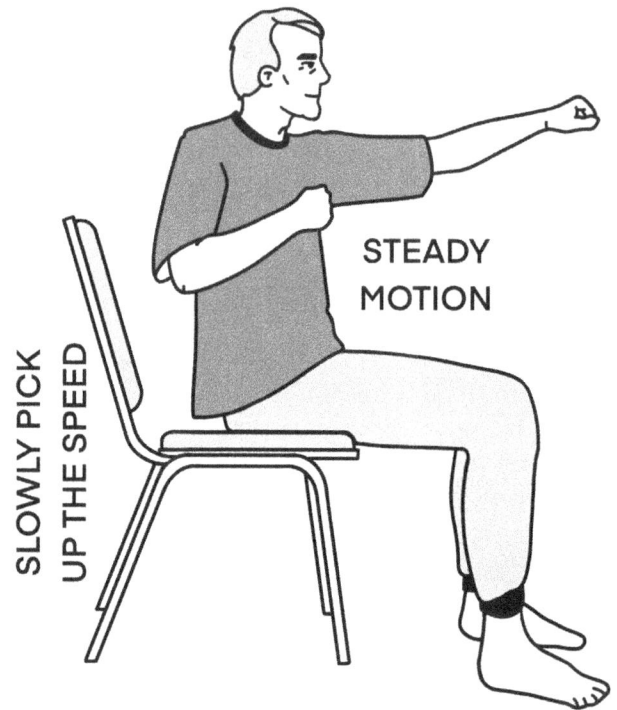

SLOWLY PICK UP THE SPEED

STEADY MOTION

SEATED SKATERS

Focus: Elevates the heart rate, improves coordination, and engages the glutes and core.

- Sit tall toward the edge of the chair with your feet flat on the floor.

- Extend your right leg diagonally to the side while reaching both arms across your body to the left as if you are skating.

- Return to the starting position and alternate sides. Pick up the speed as you get comfortable with the movement.

- Perform for 30 seconds.

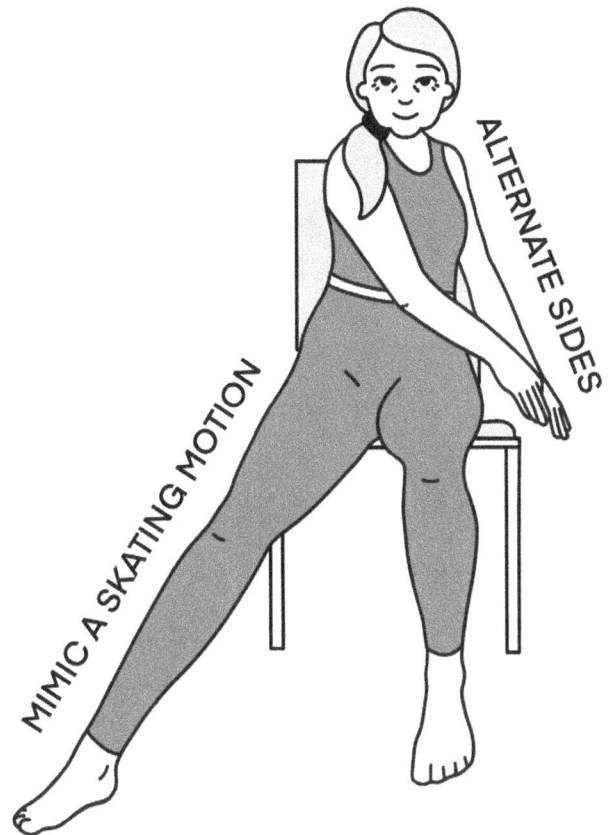

MIMIC A SKATING MOTION

ALTERNATE SIDES

SEATED RUNNING

Focus: Increases cardiovascular endurance and coordination.

- Sit tall with your feet flat on the floor toward the edge of the chair.

- Lift one knee toward your chest while lifting the opposite arm. Imagine the motion of running in one spot. Keep alternating sides as fast as you can without compromising your form. Pick up the speed, if possible.

- Perform for 30 seconds.

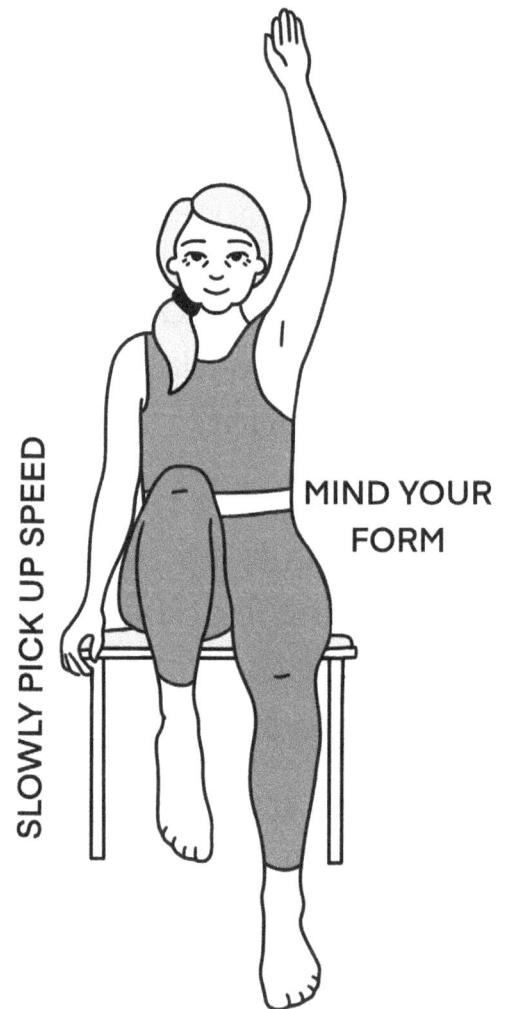

SLOWLY PICK UP SPEED

MIND YOUR FORM

SEATED JUMP ROPE

Focus: Improves cardiovascular endurance, coordination, and upper body strength.

- Sit tall and come to the balls of your feet.

- Pretend you are holding a jump rope; slightly raise your arms by your sides with loose fists.

- Begin circling your wrists as if swinging a rope while lightly bouncing your feet off the ground. Keep a steady rhythm, and increase the speed, if possible.

- Perform for 30 seconds.

KEEP STEADY RHYTHM

ENGAGE CORE

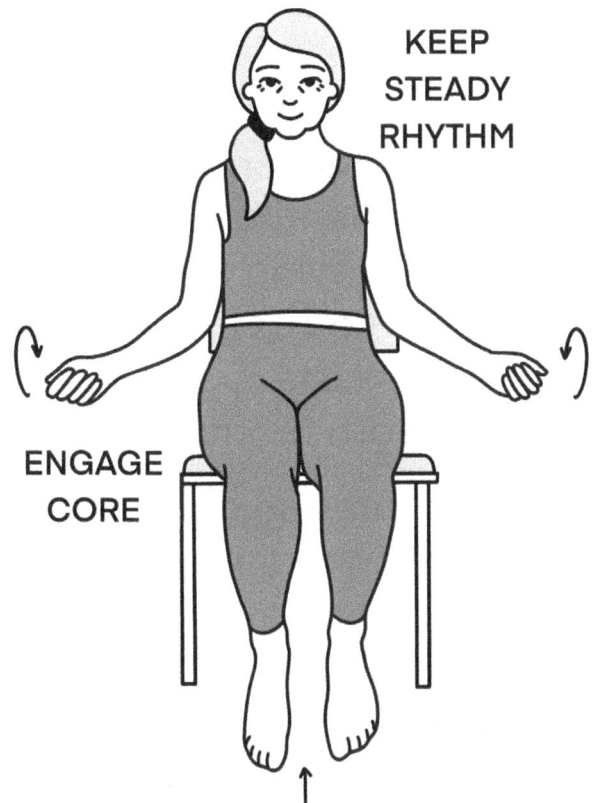

These exercises are a fun and low-impact way to incorporate movements that benefit your heart health into your routine. In the next chapter, we discuss how we can adapt and modify the exercises we've discussed so far. This is important to increase comfort and to cater to individuals who might be dealing with specific conditions.

SETTING AND ACHIEVING GOALS

10

Although it is common to lose motivation, it has been well-documented that setting a specific goal has a positive effect on staying focused and maintaining regular physical activity. If you set realistic goals, they can motivate you to stay consistent on your journey to better fitness, and provide both motivation and a sense of purpose.

Having a precise goal will help you visualize what you are working toward. Plus, the structured 4-week chair exercise program will make it even easier to stay on track to achieve your goal. There is no need to think about what workout you should do every day, the plan is laid out for you.

Goals also help you track progress and celebrate achievements. If you complete a program without having set a goal, how would you be able to measure how far you have come? It's important to set a goal so that you keep yourself accountable along your fitness journey. Then, when you reach the end of a program, you can reflect on your goal and celebrate the achievements you have made.

HOW TO SET SMART GOALS

Now that we understand why setting a goal is important, let's dive into the how.

We recommend using the SMART criteria for setting your goal for the 4-week chair exercise program. This is a well-known framework used within many disciplines to establish an effective and realistic goal.

The SMART acronym stands for:

S=Specific   **M**=Measurable   **A**=Achievable

R=Relevant   **T**=Time-bound

Here is an example of what a SMART goal could look like in the context of the 4-week chair exercise program presented in this book:

"By the end of 4 weeks, I will improve my ability to stand from a chair unassisted and increase my walking distance."

The goal is specific, time-bound, and relevant: it will help you work on your daily functional fitness and maintain your independence in a measurable way.

Specific: You will improve your lower body strength, balance, and cardiovascular endurance.

Measurable: You can measure improvement using the 30-second sit-to-stand test and the 2-minute step test (see self-assessment tests in the next section).

Achievable: You can attain your goal by using the structure of the 4-week chair exercise program.

Relevant: Your goal aligns with a valuable plan to improve your overall physical health and functional fitness.

Time-Bound: You set a specific time frame of 4 weeks to accomplish the goal.

Your SMART goal will not look exactly like this one and that is perfectly fine. Everyone is at a different point in their fitness journey and goals should be tailored to each person.

Try to dive deep into what your needs are currently as you set your goal. What aspect or aspects of your health need the most attention or improvement at the moment? The SMART structure is there to guide you and to make sure the goal you establish is attainable and specific to you.

METHODS FOR TRACKING PROGRESS

Below are different methods you can use to track your progress along your fitness journey.

Keep a journal: Use a journal to record exercises, repetitions, and sets. Make note of your perceived effort on each day of performing the chair exercise program. You could rate your effort on a scale of 1-10; 10 being the most difficult effort you ever had to do. Or, keep it simple by writing down if the exercise session was easy, medium, or difficult.

If you are consistently in the easy zone, try to increase the intensity a little by adding more resistance or repetitions. However, if you're always in the difficult zone, try to dial it back so that you don't burn out.

Get some feedback: Get feedback from yourself or the people surrounding you. Reflect weekly on whether exercises feel easier or if you notice changes in daily activities, such as standing up more easily or more ease with walking. Ask loved ones if they have noticed any changes in how you move or walk. If there is a specific movement you wish to improve, you could ask someone to take a before and after video to see if there is a difference in how it's performed.

Re-Assess your fitness: Perform the fitness tests provided in the section below after completing the 4-week chair exercise program. This is a great way to compare your fitness level before putting in the work and after. It takes about 4 weeks to start seeing changes in fitness levels when undertaking a program. Therefore, re-assessing your abilities after the 4-week program is a good time frame.

ADJUST GOALS AS NEEDED

Sometimes you need to adjust our goal to make it fit your realistic needs. This might mean that you need to make it easier, or more challenging. Here are some tips to retarget your goal as you move through your fitness challenge:

Change in physical condition: If your physical condition changes during the 4-week chair exercise program, make sure you adjust your goal accordingly. Don't be afraid to dial it back if needed.

Adjust goal intensity: If you reach your goal before you finish the 4-week chair exercise program, modify your goal to create a new challenge for yourself. On the other hand, if you are struggling through the 4-week program and realize your goal is unrealistic, it may be necessary to reframe it.

Revise the timeline to attain your goal: If progress is slower than expected, you could also allow yourself more time to complete the 4-week chair exercise program. Instead of reaching your goal in 4 weeks, it might take you 6 weeks to attain it, and that is alright.

Focus on the journey: Sometimes, we need to focus on what we accomplish on a day-to-day basis, instead of only thinking about the result. While your end goal is important, try to notice and celebrate your everyday achievements. If you had a good workout on a given day, take time to be proud of yourself for showing up. Trust that if you stay consistent, you will get great results.

STAYING MOTIVATED AND OVERCOMING CHALLENGES 11

Setbacks happen to everyone; it's part of any fitness journey. The reality is, that sometimes life gets in the way of our goals. If you miss a day or two, don't be discouraged. What's important is to start again and keep moving forward. To help you deal with setbacks, here are a few tips to remember:

Change your mindset: Try to look at your progress as a long-term concept instead of trying to achieve perfection every single day. Missing one or two days of workouts or struggling with a specific workout doesn't erase all the hard work you accomplished in the past. Pick up where you left off and keep going.

Use positive self-talk: When we have bad days or get derailed from our goals, it's easy to fall into the trap of being mean to ourselves. Speak to yourself with compassion as you would to a friend who is feeling discouraged. Avoid negative self-talk like "I can't do this" or "I'm not good enough." Instead, use phrasing like "I'm doing my best, and that is enough" or "I can do hard things."

Reconnect with your goal: Read your goal again to remind yourself why you decided to start this program. Was it to feel stronger? Was it to be able to walk for longer distances? Whatever it may be, keeping your eyes on the prize can help you stay motivated and push through setbacks.

Adjust your program as needed: We touched on this aspect when discussed that goals may need to be adjusted along the way. Sometimes, setbacks happen because the program feels too challenging. Remember that it's perfectly acceptable to modify your strategy. Decrease the challenge by reducing the number of sets or repetitions you perform or taking more breaks between each exercise.

TIPS FOR MAINTAINING A ROUTINE

The best way to create a new habit is to integrate it into your daily routine. To keep the momentum going, try these three tricks:

Schedule your workouts: Treat your workout session like it's an appointment you can't miss.

Use visual reminders: Print out the 4-Week Chair Exercise Program and post it where you will be able to see it regularly. This will provide a daily reminder to workout.

Reward yourself: Reward yourself for your effort. For example, after completing a week of workouts, treat yourself to something you enjoy to reinforce the idea that working toward your goals is worth celebrating.

HOW TO ASSESS DISCOMFORT

Discomfort and pain are not the same. Some discomfort is normal when stretching a muscle. Some light burning sensation is also normal when strengthening a muscle with resistance. Remember that experiencing pain at an intensity of 3 on a scale of 1-10 is in the safe zone. If the pain intensifies, or if you experience sudden sharp or persistent pain, pause and reassess. Decide if you need to modify the exercise, or if you should skip the exercise entirely. Don't hesitate to speak with your healthcare provider if the pain persists.

FINDING MOTIVATION THROUGH COMMUNITY

Even though chair exercises are typically done in the comfort of your own home, this doesn't mean you can't involve others. You could join an online community to discuss your progress on this journey. This is a great way to stay motivated and see what other like-minded individuals are going through.

Another way to engage with others is to involve friends or family members. Tell them about the program you are undertaking. Some may even want to take on the challenge at the same time as you. If nothing else, it's a good idea to let others know what you are doing so they can keep you accountable.

How can we properly engage with others to stay motivated on our fitness journey? Here are a few tips that might be helpful:

Share your journey: Post updates or progress in an online community group or by sending messages to friends. This might be inspiring for others and they can give you positive feedback. This can be a strong motivating factor to keep pushing you forward.

Learn from others: Swap tips, modifications, or favorite exercises with friends or fellow community members.

Celebrate together: Reaching milestones is even better when you can share it with people who are closest to you. Try to surround yourself with people who are positive and lift you up.

4-WEEK CHAIR EXERCISE PROGRAM

12

Welcome to the 4-Week Chair Exercise Program! This program is designed to help you improve your strength, flexibility, balance, and cardiovascular fitness, all while using a chair. It is meant to be safe, enjoyable, and easy to follow in the comfort of your own home. Here are the main goals you can expect to attain after completing this program:

- You can expect to feel stronger, more flexible, and more confident in performing your daily activities.

- You may also notice changes in your stamina like walking longer distances or going up and down stairs more easily.

- Finally, we hope that you find this program provides positive psychological changes. Some examples include less stress or less fear of falling.

Below is the structure this program will be following each week:

- Each week includes four 20-minute workouts.

- Two workouts will be more strength-focused and the two others will be more balance and flexibility-focused. Some cardio will be sprinkled into each workout.

- Every session includes a warm-up, cardio, and cool-down.

- We recommend also including 150 minutes of light to moderate activity like walking, swimming, or dancing each week.

- The greyed-out zones in the table are rest days from the chair exercises.

WEEK 1-2: BUILDING THE FOUNDATION

Week 1 | Goal: Activate all muscle groups with gentle movement.

WARM UP

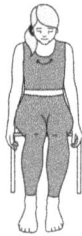

Neck rolls
10 reps

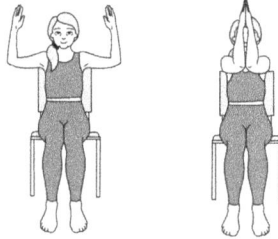

Seated chest opener
10 reps

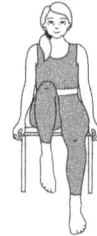

Seated marches
10 reps

WORKOUT

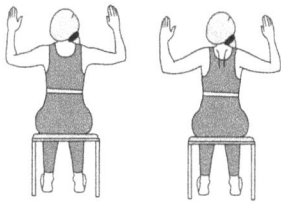

Shoulder blade squeezes
Hold for 10 sec x 5

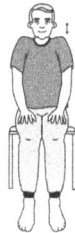

Shoulder shrugs
Hold for 10 sec x 5

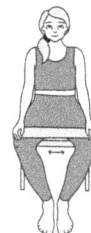

Clams
10 reps x 2

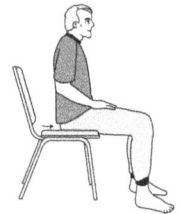

Glute squeeze
Hold for 10 sec x 5

COOL-DOWN

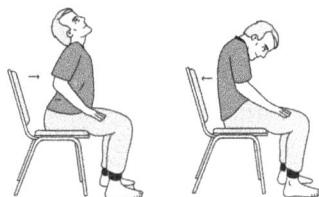

Seated cat-cow stretch
Hold for 30 sec x 2

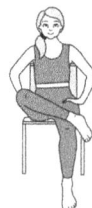

Figure-4 stretch
Hold for 30 sec x 2

Week 1 | Goal: Activate all muscle groups with gentle movement.

DAY 2 - REST

DAY 3

WARM UP

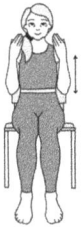

**Bending &
extending elbows**
10 reps

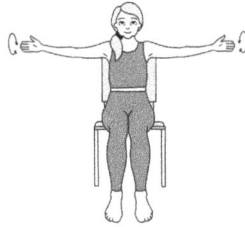

Arm circles
10 reps

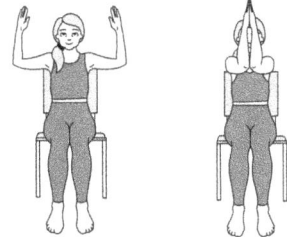

Seated chest opener
10 reps

WORKOUT

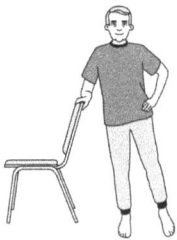

Weight shifts
10 reps x 2

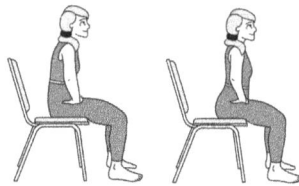

Pelvic tilts
10 reps x 2

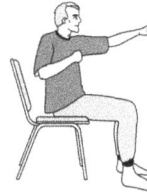

Seated punches
Hold for 30 sec x 2

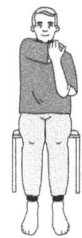

**Cross-body
arm stretch**
Hold for 30 sec x 2

COOL-DOWN

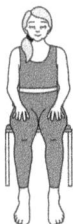

Box breathing
2-3 minutes

DAY 4 - REST

DAY 5

WARM UP

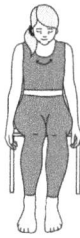

Neck rolls
10 reps

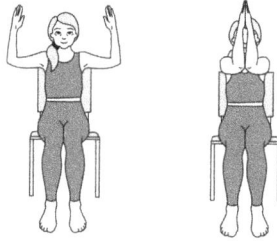

Seated chest opener
10 reps

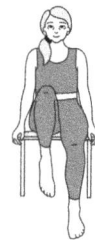

Seated marches
10 reps

WORKOUT

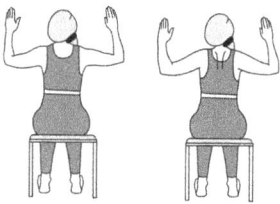

Shoulder blade squeezes
Hold for 10 sec x 5

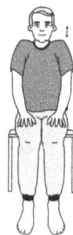

Shoulder shrugs
Hold for 10 sec x 5

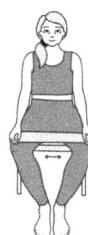

Clams
10 reps x 2

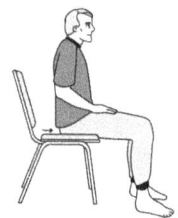

Glute squeeze
Hold for 10 sec x 5

COOL-DOWN

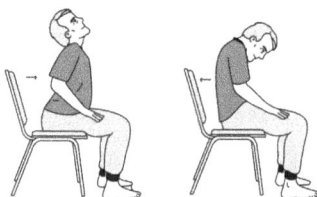

Seated cat-cow stretch
Hold for 30 sec x 2

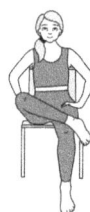

Figure-4 stretch
Hold for 30 sec x 2

Week 1 | Goal: Activate all muscle groups with gentle movement.

DAY 6 - REST

DAY 7

WARM UP

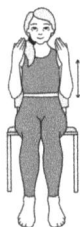

Bending & extending elbows
10 reps

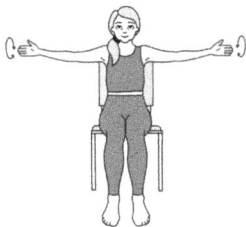

Arm circles
10 reps

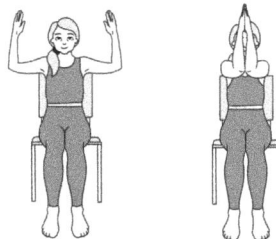

Seated chest opener
10 reps

WORKOUT

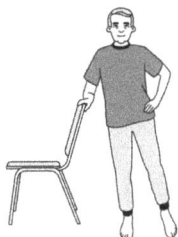

Weight shifts
10 reps x 2

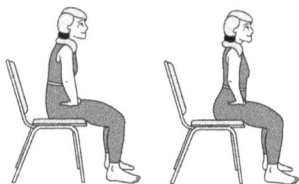

Pelvic tilts
10 reps x 2

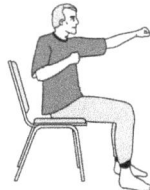

Seated punches
Hold for 30 sec x 5

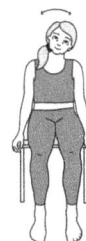

Upper trap stretch
Hold for 30 sec x 2

COOL-DOWN

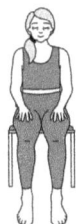

Box breathing
2-3 minutes

Week 2 | Goal: Create momentum by sticking to your routine.

DAY 1

WARM UP

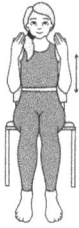

Bending & extending elbows
10 reps

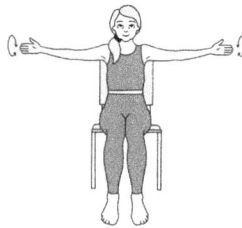

Arm circles
10 reps

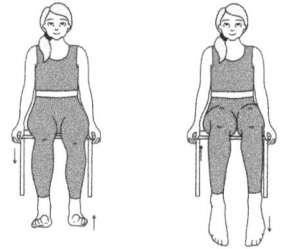

Heel-toe taps
10 reps

WORKOUT

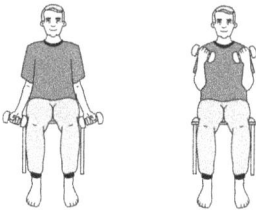

Bicep curls
10 reps x 2

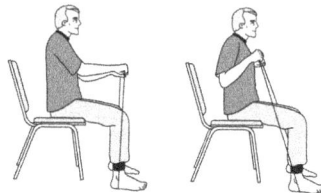

Seated rows
10 reps x 2

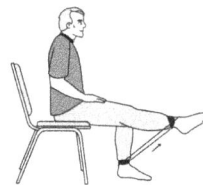

Knee extensions
10 reps x 2

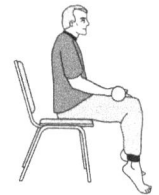

Heel Raises
10 reps x 2

COOL-DOWN

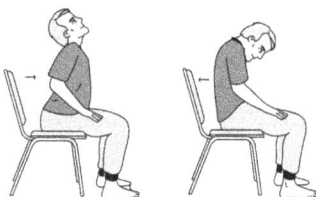

Seated cat-cow stretch
Hold 30 seconds x 2

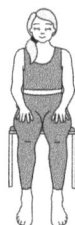

Box breathing
2-3 minutes

Week 2 | Goal: Create momentum by sticking to your routine.

DAY 2 - REST

DAY 3

WARM UP

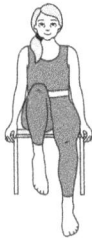

Seated marches
10 reps

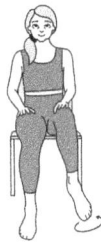

Ankle circles
10 reps

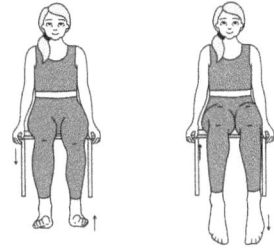

Heel-toe taps
10 reps

WORKOUT

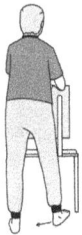

Standing side step
10 reps x 2

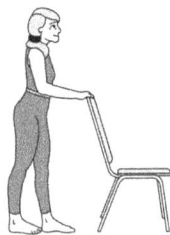

Tandem stance
30 sec/side x 2

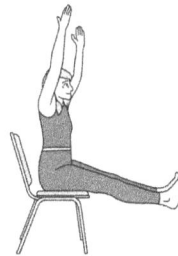

Seated jumping jacks
30 sec x 2

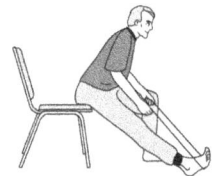

Calf stretch
Hold for 30 sec x 2

COOL-DOWN

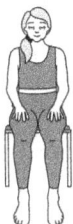

Box breathing
2-3 minutes

DAY 4 - REST

DAY 5

WARM UP

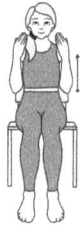

**Bending &
extending elbows**
10 reps

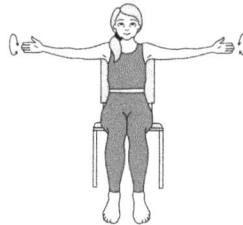

Arm circles
10 reps

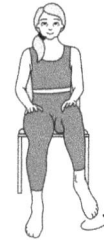

Ankle circles
10 reps

WORKOUT

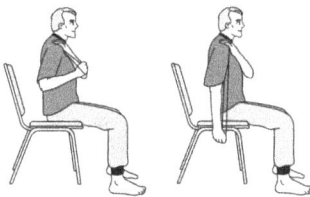

**Triceps
pull down**
10 reps x 2

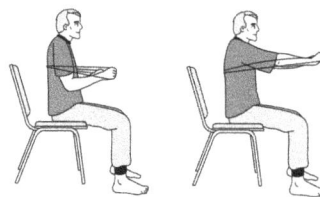

Chest presses
10 reps x 2

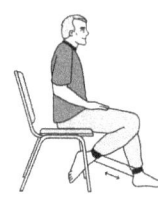

Knee flexions
10 reps x 2

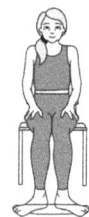

**Ankle eversions
with band**
10 reps x 2

COOL-DOWN

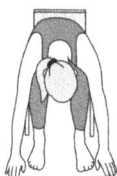

Seated forward fold
Hold for 30 seconds x 2

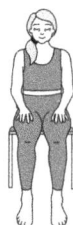

Box breathing
2-3 minutes

Week 2 | Goal: Create momentum by sticking to your routine.

DAY 6 - REST

DAY 7

WARM UP

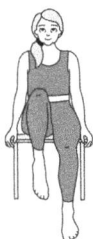

Seated marches
10 reps

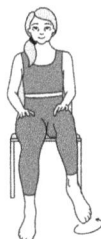

Ankle circles
10 reps

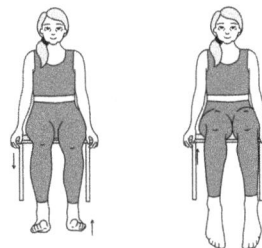

Heel-toe taps
10 reps

WORKOUT

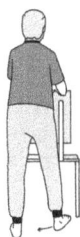

Standing side step
10 reps x 2

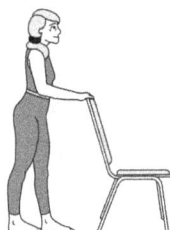

Tandem stance
30 sec/side x 2

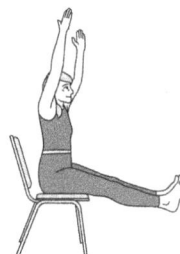

Seated jumping jacks
30 sec x 2

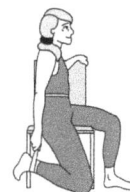

Quad stretch
Hold for 30 sec x 2

COOL-DOWN

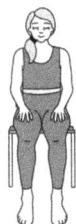

Box breathing
2-3 minutes

WEEK 3-4: BUILDING STRENGTH AND ENDURANCE

Week 3 | Goal: Challenge endurance with more core and cardio.

DAY 1

WARM UP

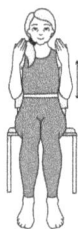

**Bending &
extending elbows**
10 reps

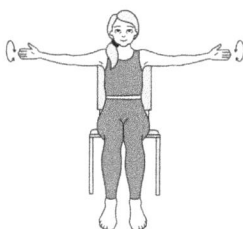

Arm circles
10 reps

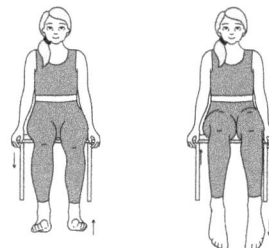

Heel-toe taps
10 reps

WORKOUT

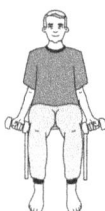

Bicep curls
10 reps x 3

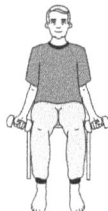

Lateral raises
10 reps x 3

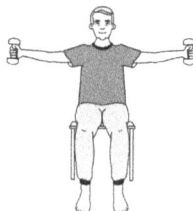

Knee extensions
10 reps x 3

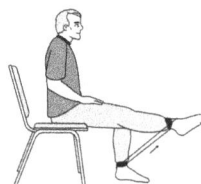

Heel Raises
15 reps x 2

COOL-DOWN

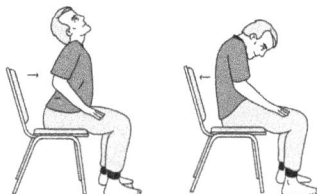

Seated cat-cow stretch
Hold for 30 seconds x2

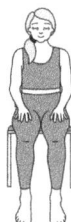

Box breathing
2-3 minutes

Week 3 | Goal: Challenge endurance with more core and cardio.

DAY 2 - REST

DAY 3

WARM UP

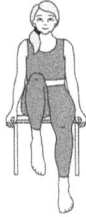

Seated marches
10 reps

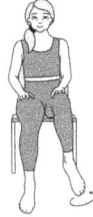

Ankle circles
10 reps

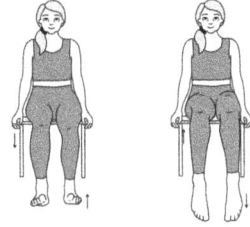

Heel-toe taps
10 reps

WORKOUT

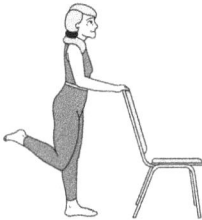

One-legged stance
30 sec/side x 2

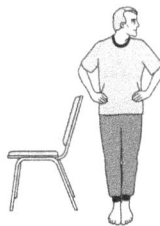

**Narrow stance
with neck rotation**
10 reps x 2

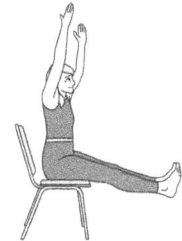

**Seated
jumping jacks**
30 sec x 2

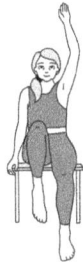

Seated running
30 sec x 5

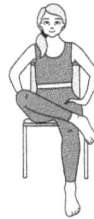

Figure-4 stretch
Hold for 30 sec x 2

COOL-DOWN

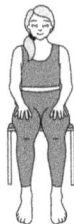

Box breathing
2-3 minutes

DAY 4 - REST

DAY 5

WARM UP

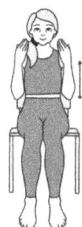

**Bending &
extending elbows**
10 reps

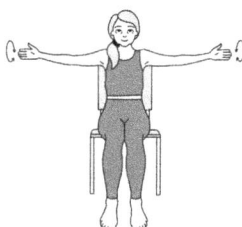

Arm circles
10 reps

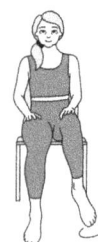

Ankle circles
10 reps

WORKOUT

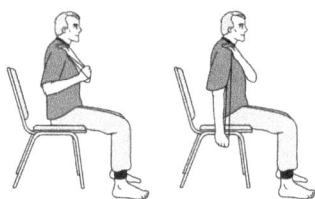

Triceps pull down
10 reps x 3

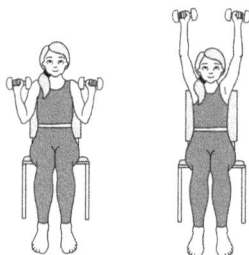

Shoulder presses
10 reps x 2

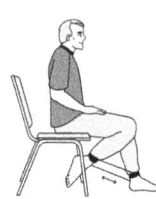

Knee flexions
10 reps x 3

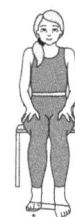

Toe taps
10 reps x 2

COOL-DOWN

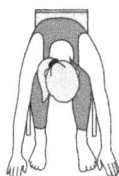

Seated forward fold
Hold for 30 seconds x 2

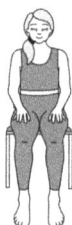

Box breathing exercise
2-3 minutes

Week 3 | Goal: Challenge endurance with more core and cardio.

DAY 6 - REST

DAY 7

WARM UP

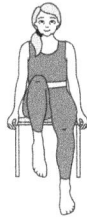

Seated marches
10 reps

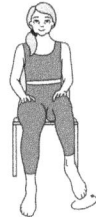

Ankle circles
10 reps

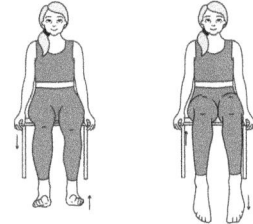

Heel-toe taps
10 reps

WORKOUT

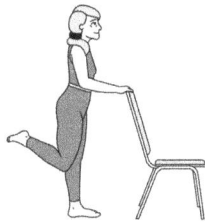

One-legged stance
30 sec/side x 2

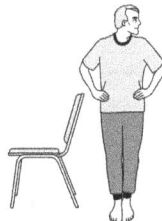

**Narrow stance
with neck rotation**
10 reps x 2

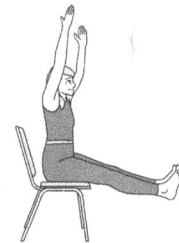

**Seated
jumping jacks**
30 sec x 2

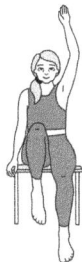

Seated running
30 sec x 5

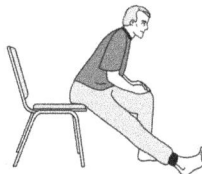

Hamstring stretch
Hold for 30 sec x 2

COOL-DOWN

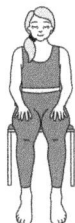

Box breathing exercise
2-3 minutes

Week 4 | Goal: Increase intensity to increase stamina.

DAY 1

WARM UP

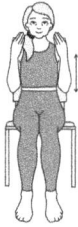

Bending & extending elbows
10 reps

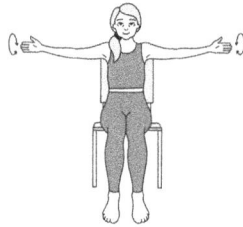

Arm circles
10 reps

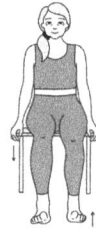

Heel-toe taps
10 reps

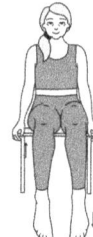

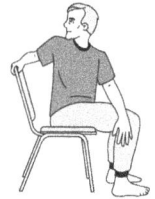

Seated twist
10 reps

WORKOUT

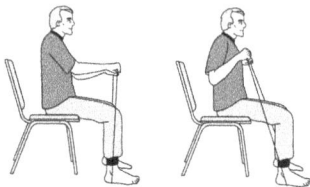

Seated rows
10 reps x 3

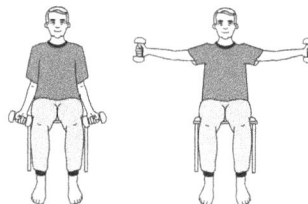

Lateral raises
10 reps x 2

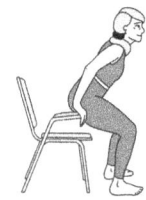

Assisted squats
10 reps x 2

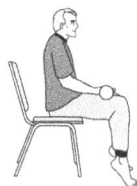

Heel raises
15 reps x 2

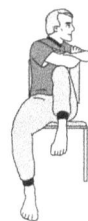

Oblique twists
10 reps x 2

COOL-DOWN

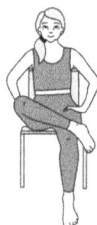

Figure-4 stretch
Hold for 30 sec x 2

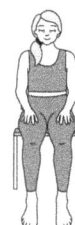

Box breathing
2-3 minutes

Week 4 | Goal: Increase intensity to increase stamina.

DAY 2 - REST

DAY 3

WARM UP

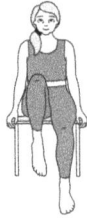

Seated marches
10 reps

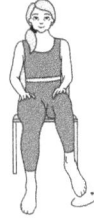

Ankle circles
10 reps

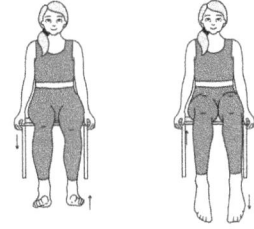

Heel-toe taps
10 reps

WORKOUT

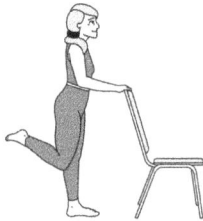

One-legged stance
30 sec/side x 2

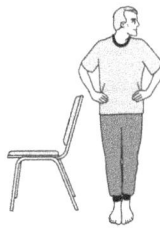

**Narrow stance
with neck rotation**
15 reps x 2

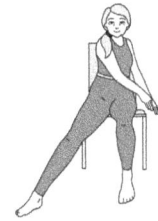

Seated skaters
30 sec x 5

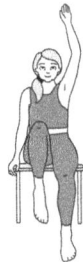

Seated running
30 sec x 5

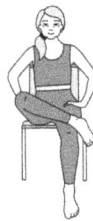

Figure-4 stretch
Hold for 30 sec x 2

COOL-DOWN

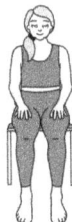

Box breathing
2-3 minutes

Week 4 | Goal: Increase intensity to increase stamina.

DAY 4 - REST
DAY 5

WARM UP

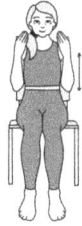

Bending & extending elbows
10 reps

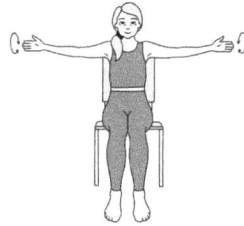

Arm circles
10 reps

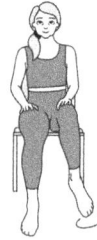

Ankle circles
10 reps

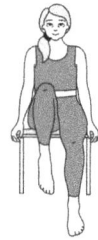

Seated marches
10 reps

WORKOUT

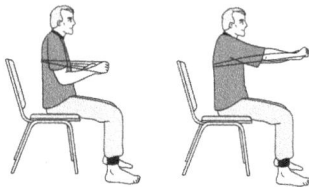

Chest presses
10 reps x 2

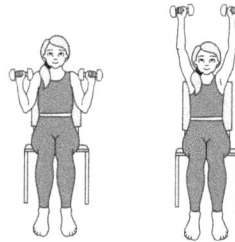

Shoulder presses
10 reps x 2

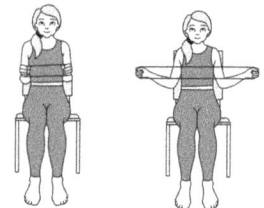

External rotation of the shoulder
10 reps x 2

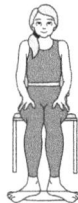

Ankle eversions with a band
10 reps x 2

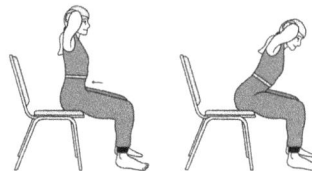

Abdominal crunch
10 reps x 2

COOL-DOWN

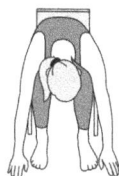

Seated forward fold
Hold for 30 seconds x 2

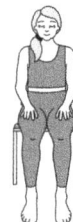

Box breathing
2-3 minutes

Week 4 | Goal: Increase intensity to increase stamina.

DAY 6 - REST
DAY 7

WARM UP

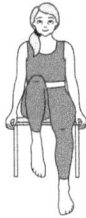

Seated marches
10 reps

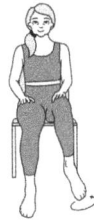

Ankle circles
10 reps

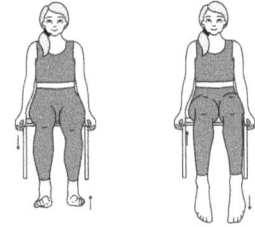

Heel-toe taps
10 reps

WORKOUT

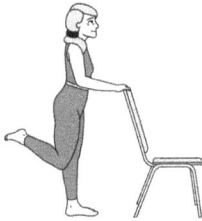

One-legged stance
30 sec/side x 2

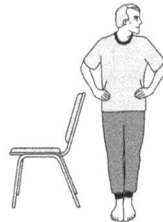

**Narrow stance
with neck rotation**
10 reps x 2

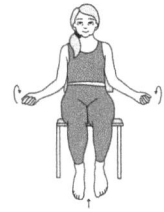

**Seated jump
rope**
30 sec x 5

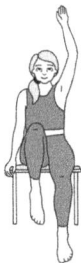

Seated running
30 sec x 5

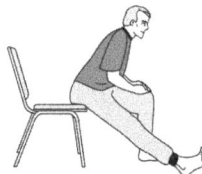

Hamstring stretch
Hold for 30 sec x 2

COOL-DOWN

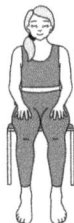

Box breathing
2-3 minutes

CONGRATULATIONS

You've reached the end of the *Move Better, Feel Better Chair Exercises for Seniors Over 60* program, but now is the time to keep going! Establishing a routine is often the hardest step. Like most aspects of health, exercise is a continuous journey. Keep integrating these chair exercises into your fitness routine and revisit this book as needed.

Know that this journey should be about more than just physical fitness. It's also about building confidence, staying active, and finding joy in movement.

Celebrate every small victory, stay connected with your goals and community, and most importantly, enjoy the process. You've got this!

REFERENCES

Afonso, J., et al. Revisiting the 'Whys' and 'Hows' of the Warm-Up: Are We Asking the Right Questions? Sports Medicine. 54.1 (2024): 23–30. https://doi.org/10.1007/s40279-023-01908-y

Afonso, J., Olivares-Jabalera, J., & Andrade, R. Time to Move From Mandatory Stretching? We Need to Differentiate "Can I?" From "Do I Have To?" Frontiers in Physiology. (2021)12. https://doi.org/10.3389/fphys.2021.714166

Bohannon, R. W., & Crouch, R. H. Two-Minute Step Test of Exercise Capacity: Systematic Review of Procedures, Performance, and Clinimetric Properties. Journal of Geriatric Physical Therapy 42.2 (2019):105–112. https://doi.org/10.1519/JPT.0000000000000164

Chilibeck, P. D., et al. Evidence-based risk assessment and recommendations for physical activity: arthritis, osteoporosis, and low back pain. Applied Physiology, Nutrition, and Metabolism. 36.S1 (2011): S49–S79. https://doi.org/10.1139/h11-037

de Souza, I. et al. Prevalence of low back pain in the elderly population: a systematic review. Clinics. 74 (2019): e789. https://doi.org/10.6061/clinics/2019/e789

Garstang, K. R., et al. What Effect Do Goal Setting Interventions Have on Physical Activity and Psychological Outcomes in Insufficiently Active Adults? A Systematic Review and Meta-Analysis. Journal of Physical Activity & Health, 21.6 (2024): 541–553. https://doi.org/10.1123/jpah.2023-0340

Kang KY. Effects of core muscle stability training on the weight distribution and stability of the elderly. J Phys Ther Sci. 10 (27 October 2015):3163-5. doi: 10.1589/jpts.27.3163.

Keller, K., & Engelhardt, M. Strength and muscle mass loss with aging process. Age and strength loss. Muscles, Ligaments and Tendons Journal. 3.4 (2014): 346–350.

Klempel, N., et al. The Effect of Chair-Based Exercise on Physical Function in Older Adults: A Systematic Review and Meta-Analysis. International Journal of Environmental Research and Public Health. 18.4 (2021): 1902. https://doi.org/10.3390/ijerph18041902

La Greca, S., et al. Acute and Chronic Effects of Supervised Flexibility Training in Older Adults: A Comparison of Two Different Conditioning Programs. International Journal of Environmental Research and Public Health. 19.24 (2022): 16974. https://doi.org/10.3390/ijerph192416974

Mackie, P., & Eng, J. J. The influence of seated exercises on balance, mobility, and cardiometabolic health outcomes in individuals living with a stroke: A systematic review and meta-analysis. Clinical Rehabilitation. 37.7 (2023): 927–941. https://doi.org/10.1177/02692155221150002

Madhushri, P., et al. A Health Tool Suite for Mobility Assessment. Inf. 7 (2016): 47.

Magutah, K., Thairu, K., & Patel, N. Effect of short moderate intensity exercise bouts on cardiovascular function and maximal oxygen consumption in sedentary older adults. BMJ Open Sport & Exercise Medicine. 6.1 (2020): e000672. https://doi.org/10.1136/bmjsem-2019-000672

McGowan, C. J., Pyne, D. B., Thompson, K. G., & Rattray, B. Warm-Up Strategies for Sport and Exercise: Mechanisms and Applications. Sports Medicine. 45.11 (2015): 1523–1546. https://doi.org/10.1007/s40279-015-0376-x

National Institute on Aging. (n.d.). Heart Health and Aging. U.S. Department of Health and Human Services. https://www.nia.nih.gov/health/heart-health/heart-health-and-aging

O'Sullivan, S. B., Schmitz, T. J., & Fulk, G. D. Physical Rehabilitation (6th ed.). F. A. Davis Company, 2014.

Platz, K., Kools, S., & Howie-Esquivel, J. Benefits, Facilitators, and Barriers of Alternative Models of Cardiac Rehabilitation: A QUALITATIVE SYSTEMATIC REVIEW. Journal of Cardiopulmonary Rehabilitation and Prevention. 43.2 (2023): 83–92. https://doi.org/10.1097/HCR.0000000000000738

Ramsey, K. A., et al. The association of objectively measured physical activity and sedentary behavior with skeletal muscle strength and muscle power in older adults: A systematic review and meta-analysis. Aging Research Reviews, 67 (2021): 101266. https://doi.org/10.1016/j.arr.2021.101266

Rikli, R.E. and Jones, C.J. Functional Fitness Normative Scores for Community Residing Older Adults Ages 60-94. Journal of Aging and Physical Activity. 7 (1999): 160-179. https://doi.org/10.1123/japa.7.2.162

Rikli, R.E. and Jones, C.J. Measuring functional fitness of older adults. The Journal on Active Aging, March/April (2002): 24–30.

Van Hooren, B., & Peake, J. M. Do We Need a Cool-Down After Exercise? A Narrative Review of the Psychophysiological Effects and the Effects on Performance, Injuries and the Long-Term Adaptive Response. Sports Medicine. 48.7 (2018): 1575–1595. https://doi.org/10.1007/s40279-018-0916-2

Wang, J., Li, Y., Yang, G. Y., & Jin, K. Age-Related Dysfunction in Balance: A Comprehensive Review of Causes, Consequences, and Interventions. Aging and Disease. (2024). https://doi.org/10.14336/AD.2024.0124-1

BONUS THANK YOU

Thank you for choosing **Move Better, Feel Better Chair Exercises for Seniors Over 60**. We hope this book has provided you with the guidance and inspiration needed for your wellness journey. Your commitment to improving your health and well-being is truly commendable. Remember, every small step you take brings you closer to a healthier, happier you. Keep going, and stay motivated!

Don't forget to claim your bonus. Go to your internet browser and type in **https://www.getmovefit.com/chairexercisesbonus** to register for the unlimited and free portal access. There are no hidden extra costs, this is completely free with the purchase of this book.

The PIN code to unlock your bonus is **15135**

These bonuses are **FREE** and designed to **help you achieve your goals**.

With gratitude,
Linette Cunley

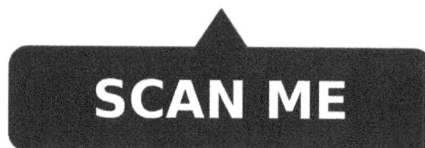

SCAN ME

www.ingramcontent.com/pod-product-compliance
Lightning Source LLC
Chambersburg PA
CBHW080001280326
41935CB00013B/1708